DEFEATING CANCER

PHILIP A. SALEM, M.D.
WITH DENNY ANGELLE

DEFEATING CANCER

KNOWLEDGE ALONE IS NOT ENOUGH

QUARTET BOOKS

First published in 2018 by Quartet Books Limited
A member of the Namara Group
27 Goodge Street, London, W1T 2LD

A catalogue record for this book is available from the British Library

ISBN 9780704374522

Text design and typesetting by Tetragon, London
Printed and bound in Great Britain by T J International Ltd, Padstow, Cornwall

To my wife, Wadad, and my children,
Dara, Khaled and Rayya.

CONTENTS

Disclaimers   ix

Acknowledgments   xi

About the Author   xiii

Preface   xvii

PART I: A LETTER TO THE CANCER PATIENT

1 Diagnosis   3

2 Staging   15

3 The Group Consultation   27

4 Preparing for Treatment   39

5 Surgery: A Medical Oncologist's Perspective   50

6 Radiation Therapy: A Medical Oncologist's Perspective   56

7 Radiation Therapy: A Radiation Oncologist's Perspective   63

8 Systemic Therapy   70

9 Medical Supportive Therapy   83

10 The Power of Hope, Perseverance, Love and Compassion   94

11 Quality of Life   103

PART II: ESSAYS ON MEDICAL PRACTICE AND THE RIGHT TO HEALTH

12 The Power of Education   113

13 Telling the Truth   122

14 The Impact of Insurance and Regulatory Oversight
    on Medicine   132

15 Health as a Human Right   143

Afterword   147

Citations   149

DISCLAIMERS

This book is intended as an informational and educational resource for cancer patients and their families. It should not be considered medical advice and does not replace professional medical care. Some of the recommendations made here are the opinions of the author and should not be interpreted as statements on standards of care. Every patient and family is unique. This book should not be considered applicable to every patient or family. Physicians should exercise their best clinical judgment in the care of each individual patient and family. The author has made every effort to ensure the accuracy and timeliness of the information contained in this book, but medical science and cancer treatments advance rapidly with new information constantly emerging. Patients and families with concerns about cancer, cancer risk or other medical conditions should seek care from a qualified medical professional.

The case stories included in this book are intended to illustrate important points and messages. Names have been changed and certain details have been altered to protect patient confidentiality.

The quotations included in this book are intended to complement the message of the text. Except for quotations by Dr. Philip Salem and Dr. Bin Teh, the quotations used were pulled from publicly available resources that are cited with each quotation. The individuals or groups to whom the quotations are attributed have not been contacted to confirm the accuracy of the quotations, nor have they given their permission for the inclusion of the quotations in this book. No association of any kind should be inferred between the quoted individuals or groups and this book and its contents.

ACKNOWLEDGMENTS

Writing this book has long been a goal of mine. It is the result of my many years of experience in cancer medicine, but I could not have achieved it without the help of many people.

To my patients, I offer my sincere gratitude and respect. I have learned so much from you over these many years. You have taught me about hope, love, compassion and perseverance. You have shown me the strength and power of the human spirit and the importance of living a good life. It has been my great honor to travel with you on your journeys with cancer. You are my inspiration for this book, and I have written every chapter with you in mind.

To all the remarkable people I have worked with around the world throughout my career, I offer my deepest thanks. There are far too many of you to name here but without your dedication, guidance and support I would not be the physician, scientist and educator that I am today.

To my wife, Wadad, and my three amazing children, Dara, Khaled and Rayya, I give you my undying love and most humble thanks. You are the lights of my life. You encourage and support me every day and bring joy and happiness to my life.

To Dr. Bin Teh, I thank you for your chapter on radiation therapy. Your perspectives as a radiation oncologist have been invaluable to me over the years and your chapter will be of great value to readers of this book.

To Dr. Raye Alford of Genetics Genomics Consulting LLC, I thank you for your assistance with writing and preparing this book. You have taken my thoughts and ideas and assembled them into this book of which I am so proud.

To Dr. Lois DeBakey, I thank you for connecting me with Denny Angelle and Dr. Alford. Without you, this book would never have come into being.

And finally, to my readers, I thank you for your time and interest. It is my sincere hope that you and your loved ones find this book to be informative and educational, and that it gives you support and guidance as you embark on your journey to fight cancer.

ABOUT THE AUTHOR

Philip Adib Salem, M.D. is a world-renowned cancer physician, researcher, educator, author and international medical statesman. He was born in Bterram, El-Koura, North Lebanon, in 1941. Guided by his parents' passion for education, discipline and hard work, he earned his Doctor of Medicine degree from the School of Medicine of the American University of Beirut in Beirut, Lebanon in 1965. He completed his residency and fellowship training at the American University of Beirut Medical Center, at the Memorial Sloan Kettering Cancer Center in New York, New York, and at the M.D. Anderson Cancer Center in Houston, Texas.

Dr. Salem has treated cancer patients for more than fifty years. He served on the faculty of the American University of Beirut Medical Center as a professor of medicine and the founding director of the Cancer Research and Treatment Program from 1971 to 1987, and on the faculty of M.D. Anderson Cancer Center as a professor of cancer medicine from 1987 to 1991. In 1991, Dr. Salem was appointed director of Cancer Research at St. Luke's Episcopal Hospital in Houston, now known as the Baylor St. Luke's Medical Center, CHI St. Luke's Health, where he is currently director emeritus of Cancer Research. Also in 1991, Dr. Salem established the Salem Oncology Centre, a private cancer facility in the Texas Medical Center in Houston, where he continues to serve as president. In 2010, St. Luke's Episcopal Hospital established the Philip A. Salem Chair in Cancer Research to honor Dr. Salem's contributions to cancer medicine.

Dr. Salem has published extensively on immunoproliferative small intestinal disease and the causative relationship of infection to cancer, and on new methods he developed for delivering cancer drugs to patients to reduce toxicity and maximize efficacy. His research has also been crucial in the development of new anti-cancer agents.

Dr. Salem has served in many leadership positions over the years and was a member of a White House health care advisory committee from 1989 to 1994. He is the recipient of numerous honors and awards including honorary doctorates in Humane Letters from both the Lebanese American University and Notre Dame University of Lebanon, the Ellis Island Medal of Honor of the National Ethnic Coalition Organizations, the Khalil Gibran International Award of the Arabic Heritage League and the Solidarity Award from the Foedus Foundation, an Italian foundation for the promotion of culture, enterprise and solidarity. He was awarded the rank of Commendatore of the Order of the Merit of the Italian Republic and was listed as one of America's Top Doctors by the Castle Connolly Guide from 2001 to 2007.

Dr. Salem embraces the philosophy that, in the practice of medicine, doctors treat people, not diseases. Dr. Salem leads the struggle to re-humanize cancer treatment in America and the world. He believes that knowledge alone is not enough. Patients need love, care, hope, compassion, accessibility to the doctor and time to talk about their fears, anxieties and concerns.

Dr. Salem also champions a movement to prohibit government and insurance providers from interfering in the decision-making process for the diagnosis and treatment of cancer. He strongly believes that a doctor should have the liberty to treat patients as he or she thinks best and practice without fear of litigation for failure to comply with arbitrary standards and guidelines that may not be appropriate for every patient. Dr. Salem is also a renaissance intellectual. He has published extensively on Lebanese and Middle Eastern affairs, and has written articles on topics ranging from religion to philosophy to human rights. He advanced the concept that the most sacred human right is the right to health. Nine books have been written about him and his vision.

PREFACE

As a child, I listened to my father's stories. Every day at the dinner table, the basic theme was always the same: the power of education. Although my father had no formal education, he was the fiercest proponent for education. He felt the most important obligation he had to his children was to educate them. In my journey with learning and research, I have never met a man who was as strong an advocate for education as my father. Now, after fifty years of cancer research and medicine, I have learned how correct my father was. I have come to believe the most important weapon we have against cancer is not a drug, X-rays or surgery, it is education.

Education is why I wrote this book, which crystallizes my experience with cancer. I want to educate cancer patients about their disease and about the art and science of defeating it. I feel this book is the best gift I can give to any cancer patient because I believe the more the patient knows about his cancer and about its appropriate treatment, the better his chances are for cure.

I present this book in two parts. In the first part, I try to shepherd the cancer patient, throughout his journey with this disease, to a cure. In the second part of this book, I offer my thoughts on some of the challenges faced by doctors, patients and caregivers in the United States today. While these additional topics may seem less relevant to your journey with cancer, I hope my experience and insights, gained over years of practicing medicine, will be helpful to you.

My career in medicine began in June 1965 when I graduated from the medical school of the American University of Beirut. After medical school, I did three years of residency in internal medicine. I thought about subspecializing in kidney diseases (nephrology) until a very close friend of mine was diagnosed with ovarian cancer. I accompanied her through her journey with this brutal illness and saw how much she suffered, not only physically, with pain, but emotionally and mentally. At that time, in the mid-1960s, there was very little treatment for cancer of the ovary. Unfortunately for my friend, in addition to not being able to offer much in the way of medical treatment, her doctors also failed to listen to her concerns or show her much compassion. Her doctors never answered her questions truthfully and they left her in limbo regarding her mental and emotional agony. I watched this at a close range and decided to study oncology and to become a different kind of doctor. A doctor who cares. A doctor who listens. A doctor who does his best for his patient.

In June 1968, I started my training in cancer medicine at Memorial Sloan Kettering Cancer Center. This was the beginning of my journey with cancer. My mentor was Dr. David Karnofsky. I did two years of fellowship there and then, at the suggestion of my mentor, I traveled to Houston, Texas for a third year of fellowship in medical oncology at M.D. Anderson Cancer Center. There, my mentors were Dr. Emil Frei and Dr. Emil Freireich. It was my great fortune to study under these three founders and champions of medical oncology and to have the opportunity to train at the two most prestigious cancer centers in the world.

Since finishing my training in 1971, I have been continuously treating cancer patients and engaged in cancer research. Over the decades, I have witnessed the evolution of cancer treatment. I have learned that knowledge is fundamental to defeating cancer, but I have also learned that knowledge alone is not enough. Cancer patients also need easy access to the doctor, almost daily monitoring of disease and treatment, psychological support, hope, perseverance, love and compassion.

I believe hope and perseverance are so important to success against cancer that I have devoted a large portion of one chapter of this book to these topics. In cancer, the journey is long, and if patients decide to stop treatment, they often die. Hope and perseverance can keep patients in the fight. But hope and perseverance are not only important for the patient, they are also important for the doctor. Doctors must remember that they do not treat disease, but rather humans who have disease. The difference between these two outlooks is enormous. As a physician, I accept that if I do not treat the human who has the disease, I will not be able to give the best treatment for the disease itself. Thus, the subtitle of this book is *knowledge alone is not enough*.

I also share with you my view that the increasing intrusion of insurance systems and the ever-expanding oversight that governs the professional work of doctors have done harm to the practice of medicine. Insurance interferes in decision-making, sometimes limiting the choices a doctor can make regarding treatment. Even if you are a patient at one of the best cancer centers in America, your doctor may not be free to choose among all possible treatment options unless you can pay for certain treatments yourself. Also, doctors have become burdened by massive amounts of paperwork. A cancer patient needs a lot of time to talk to his doctor but, because of oversight, the time doctors have to talk to their patients is compromised. These are important topics because it is my belief that doctors, patients, and patient advocates must come together to defend the integrity of the doctor-patient relationship, the dignity of the patient and the right of patients to receive the best possible treatment. If we do not speak out, patients will be the victims of this assault on medicine.

In its entirety, this book is intended to help you receive the best treatment and care that you can get, and to give you the best chance for a cure. Let's begin the journey.

PHILIP A. SALEM, M.D.

PART I

A Letter to the Cancer Patient

I

Diagnosis

*Be an active partner in the medical decisions
that are made about your life!*

HAMILTON JORDAN[1]

You have just been told you have cancer. This is the beginning of your journey. You begin to feel many things. You are probably afraid. But the first thing I want you to know is that fear is your enemy. It will hinder your ability to seek the knowledge you need to get proper treatment for your cancer. It will also paralyze you when you need to make important decisions.

Is it the cancer you fear? More likely you fear the result of your cancer, the idea of suffering and the undignified journey you expect to have. You may be frightened by a shift in your sense of well-being and self-reliance. You might also be scared about the impact your cancer will have on your family.

It is natural to be afraid, but do not give in to your fear. You must get beyond your fear, so you can think rationally and make the right choices. You need to learn about your cancer and its treatment, advocate for yourself, partner with your doctors and participate in your own care. The patient who does all these things is already on the way to a cure.

∾

Know too that you are not alone. Many people are in the same situation. Many people have cancer, and many are cancer survivors. At one point in their lives, each of these people faced the truth about cancer and how it affected them.

You have many friends on this journey. Your family and friends will be with you. I too will accompany you. I have written this book because I want to shepherd you throughout this journey. So, come with me, let us take this journey together.

∾

Do you really have cancer? It may seem strange, but this is the first question for us to consider on your journey. This is your diagnosis, and it is vitally important to get it right. You cannot be treated for your cancer until you know unequivocally that you have it.

Your doctor might suspect you have cancer based on your clinical symptoms or because of a test result, but a diagnosis of cancer requires examination of a sample of tissue. It is the only way to know if you really have cancer.

If your doctor suspects you have a solid tumor, he or she will take a sample of tissue —also called a biopsy—using one or more of three approaches: fine needle aspiration biopsy, core biopsy or surgical biopsy. In a fine needle aspiration biopsy, a physician puts a needle into the mass suspected to be cancer. The needle used is very thin, and the sample taken is very small. A core biopsy is similar to a fine needle aspiration, but the needle is larger. In a core biopsy, the physician puts the needle into the suspicious mass and takes a core tissue sample. The advantage of a core biopsy is that it yields a larger sample of tissue for the doctor to examine.

Amy's story

I have known Amy for many years. Amy called me once crying. She had just been told she had breast cancer. Amy was frightened because she knew what cancer can be like. Her mother died of brain cancer, and her sister was being treated for breast cancer.

After our phone conversation, Amy came to see me. She brought her tissue samples with her. I had our pathologist examine the samples. He concluded that Amy did not have invasive cancer. Instead, he diagnosed pre-malignant lesions called ductal carcinoma *in situ* (DCIS).

The pathologist who initially reviewed Amy's samples identified DCIS but also believed he saw an area that was invasive cancer. Our pathologist disagreed.

We sought opinions from several additional pathologists. We also correlated the pathologists' diagnoses with a magnetic resonance imaging (MRI) scan of Amy's breasts and a mammogram. We determined that Amy's breasts had diffuse DCIS but everything we saw looked like DCIS, not invasive cancer. We told Amy the good news and she was relieved.

Sometimes, however, the doctor needs an even larger piece of tissue for analysis and it is necessary for the doctor to make a surgical incision to obtain the tissue required. This is a surgical biopsy.

For cancers where there is not a solid tumor to biopsy, other approaches to sample collection are used. For example, if a patient has pleural effusion (fluid around their lungs) which is thought to be due to cancer, a sample of fluid might be taken from the chest. If a patient is suspected of having a blood cancer such as leukemia, blood or bone marrow may be drawn for examination.

Sometimes more than one biopsy is needed to diagnose cancer. For example, if we do a fine needle aspiration and it is not diagnostic, which means we cannot make a certain diagnosis of cancer, then we might do a core biopsy. If that fails to lead to a definitive diagnosis a surgical biopsy might be done. It is uncommon for multiple biopsies to be needed, but it does happen. Because it is so important to have a definitive diagnosis of your cancer, perseverance is critical.

∽

The doctor who examines the sample of tissue removed by a biopsy is called a pathologist. Pathologists are very important in the diagnosis of cancer, but most people know very little about the pathologist's role.

Pathologists work in the laboratory. They may work in a hospital or for a private laboratory. A pathologist is a medical doctor (M.D.) who looks at tissues and cells through a microscope to make a diagnosis of disease. Every specialty in medicine has a corresponding specialty in pathology. Pathologists often make the initial diagnosis of cancer.

When pathologists receive a sample of tissue they take a portion of the tissue, process it and put it on glass slides to view through a microscope. The remaining tissue is put into what is called a paraffin block; paraffin is a waxy material, and this block can contain different parts of the biopsy. The tissue is placed in the paraffin in such a way that the block can be thinly sliced, exposing a cross-section of the tissue for microscopic study. Sometimes, the different sections of tissue are placed side by side for comparison.

Historically, the work of pathologists concentrated on histopathology (the microscopic study of tissues for the diagnosis of disease) and cytopathology (the microscopic study of cells isolated from body fluids, secretions or tissues for the diagnosis of disease). Histopathology and cytopathology involve looking at cells on slides and often staining the cell preparations to reveal various qualities of the cells. In the case of cancer, pathologists focus on qualities of cells characteristic of different types of cancer.

Today, however, pathologists have two powerful new tools available to them—molecular pathology and molecular genetic pathology. Molecular genetic pathology includes genetic testing. These new methods help pathologists look at cancer cells on a molecular level and allow pathologists to identify specific changes in the proteins and genes of a cancer cell, helping to understand what is going on inside the cells that make up a tumor.

Understanding the biology of a tumor is increasingly important for two reasons. First, there are more than two hundred different types of cancer. Molecular pathology and molecular genetic pathology often allow pathologists to determine exactly what type of cancer a patient has. As a result, it is frequently no longer sufficient for pathologists to use only histopathology and cytopathology to examine tissue samples. Second, many newly developed cancer treatments are designed specifically to target the unique biological characteristics of different types of cancers. In order for clinicians to select the most appropriate treatment for a patient, pathologists need to relay information to the clinician about the molecular and genetic changes that have occurred within a tumor. It is simply no longer enough for a pathologist to say "this patient has breast cancer" or "this patient has colon cancer". In many cases, the cancer needs to be analyzed at the molecular level so that the best possible treatment can be selected.

Once the pathologist has completed the examination of a biopsy specimen, he or she will make a diagnosis and send that information to the clinician who ordered the biopsy.

~

Brian's story

Brian is a young man who was being treated for carcinoma of the colon. His father had carcinoma of the colon. But when Brian came to see me we did X-rays and I discovered that his tumor was in his pancreas. I conducted a clinical evaluation and suspected this might be pancreatic cancer instead of colon cancer.

Our pathologists and blood tumor markers confirmed the diagnosis of pancreatic cancer, which changed Brian's treatment.

As a complement to a pathologist's examination of tissue samples, doctors can also use tumor markers to help with a diagnosis of cancer, especially in cases where evaluation of multiple tissue samples failed to provide a definitive diagnosis.[2]

Some tumor markers are substances, often proteins, produced by the body in response to cancer or other conditions. These substances are frequently found in blood, but tumor markers also appear in tissues or in products of the body such as urine or stool. Sometimes tumor markers are found inside a mass that a physician suspects may be cancer. Tumor markers can also be genetic changes associated with cancer. Different tumor markers are associated with different types of cancer, and many different tumor markers have been described.

Tumor markers can be very specific, making them useful in the diagnosis of cancer. Sometimes we will do a biopsy and we will see cells that could be either cancer X or cancer Y. The doctor's experience and the patient's clinical symptoms may also suggest it is probably cancer X or cancer Y. Tumor markers may resolve the uncertainty.

Caroline's story

Caroline had a mass about the size of a loaf of bread growing on her face. She had undergone three separate surgical biopsies, but the pathologists could not arrive at a diagnosis. Caroline's doctors told her the mass on her face was not cancer. Instead, they thought she might have an infection.

When I saw Caroline, I didn't believe she had an infection. The mass was continuing to grow, and it was not red, tender or painful. I suspected Caroline had cancer.

I asked Caroline to collect all her samples and bring them to me. She did, and I sent the samples to pathologists who are experts in diagnosing cancer. These pathologists confirmed Caroline had lymphoma of the bone.

Lymphoma is a type of cancer that originates in the lymphatic tissues of the body. Many organs of the body, including bone, have lymphatic tissues within them.

I treated Caroline for lymphoma and more than twelve years later she remains cancer free.

It is important to remember, however, that tumor markers can also be found in other conditions or diseases, so the detection of elevated tumor markers alone does not necessarily mean you have cancer.

David's story

David had been treated for two to three years for what was believed to be a problem with the lymph nodes in his right groin. Repeated evaluations of David's lymph nodes by pathologists failed to reveal anything diagnostic.

On his most recent visit to his doctor, David was found to also have a mass in his right pelvis. A surgical biopsy of this mass was taken. The pathologist who evaluated the specimen saw only fibrous tissue and diagnosed a desmoid tumor, a tumor of fibrous tissue which is considered benign.

What was worrisome about David's case, however, was the combination of a mass in his right pelvis and enlarged lymph nodes in his right groin. One would not expect a desmoid tumor to present in this manner. But because the surgical biopsy had revealed only fibrous tissue, I became concerned that a more invasive surgical approach would be required to reach a diagnosis.

David had surgery and the whole mass in his right pelvis was removed. Based on examination of the mass, a diagnosis of a poorly differentiated cancer of testicular origin was finally made.

I treated David for testicular cancer and he was cured.

So, do you really have cancer? The pathologist may have diagnosed cancer, but many initial pathology diagnoses are inaccurate. Tumor markers may be abnormal, but that does not necessarily mean cancer either. This is why I believe it is crucial at this stage of the cancer patient's journey to also have the clinician, preferably a medical oncologist like myself, involved in the diagnosis of cancer—the clinician has to have input. For this reason, I always say the diagnosis of cancer is a clinical pathological diagnosis.

A clinical pathological diagnosis requires that the clinician, who is looking at the patient's overall clinical picture and symptoms, and the pathologist, who is looking at the tissue samples, communicate and work together as a team to consider all the evidence and establish a diagnosis that makes scientific and medical sense. If a pathologist tells me a patient has cancer, but it doesn't look like cancer on my X-ray and on my clinical examination, I question the diagnosis. Sometimes it works the other way around—the pathologist discovers something I did not see.

The point is: the diagnosis of cancer is simply too serious to be left only to the pathologist, nor should it be left only to the clinician. The diagnosis of cancer is best achieved as a collaborative effort between clinician and pathologist—a clinical pathological diagnosis.

～

Another bit of advice I give all of my patients is to get a second opinion. After all, the important question for you is "Do I really have cancer?"

You might naturally think about a second opinion from another clinician, and that is certainly an option you may choose, but what I am talking about here is a second opinion on the pathology.

Confirm you have cancer by asking for a second opinion on your biopsy specimens. And make sure this second opinion is not

Eli's story

One day I received a call from a friend of mine who told me that his brother Eli had been diagnosed with sarcoma, a cancer of the connective tissue. My friend brought his brother to see me.

Eli had a large, hard mass in his abdomen and it indeed looked like it could be a sarcoma. I looked at Eli's medical records and found out Eli's biopsy specimens had been sent to three different institutions. All three institutions diagnosed sarcoma. But there was something in Eli's medical history that made me suspicious of this diagnosis. Eli had a low-grade fever, night sweats and itched from time to time. This was something I had seen before and I became concerned Eli might have lymphoma, not sarcoma.

I sent Eli's pathology specimens to another pathologist—one who is a world-renowned expert in lymphoma. He diagnosed lymphoma. Subsequently, the pathologist who originally made the diagnosis of sarcoma reexamined the samples more thoroughly and agreed this was, in fact, lymphoma.

I treated Eli for lymphoma and he made a full recovery.

just from any pathologist but one who has a lot of experience in diagnosing cancer. If you live in a small city or town, you may wish to seek a second opinion from a pathologist at a large cancer center. You may have to be persistent, but your physician should be able to find a pathologist with experience in diagnosing cancer to provide a second opinion.

Getting a second opinion on your biopsy specimens is important because, even in America where the best medical care in the world is available, many patients do not receive the most appropriate treatment for their cancer. Your chances of achieving the best possible outcome depend upon receiving proper treatment. But you cannot receive proper treatment if you do not have an accurate and detailed diagnosis of your cancer. Getting a second opinion from an expert pathologist can help you and your doctor to be confident that you are headed in the right direction as you take your next steps on this journey.

At this point I want to remind you that cancer does not occur overnight. It takes time. By the time a patient comes to the doctor with symptoms of cancer it is likely the cancer has been there for many years. The reason I say this is to remind you to slow down. Cancer is not an emergency. There is never an urgency to treat cancer the next day. Of course, there are emergencies in cancer care, but the diagnosis itself is never an emergency.

Do things in a disciplined and rational manner, not a passionate or rushed manner. Educate yourself. Establish a dialogue with your doctor. Participate in your care. Take the time to get a second opinion on your diagnosis of cancer, even a third opinion, if you can.

Making a definitive, unequivocal diagnosis is the first step and a strategic milestone in your journey. It may take a little time, but it is time well spent.

∼

Now that you are certain you have cancer, and you know exactly what type of cancer you have, let's move on to the second step in your journey: staging your cancer.

2

STAGING

Diagnosis is not the end, but the beginning of practice.

MARTIN H. FISCHER, M.D.[1]

After diagnosis comes the next step in your journey: staging your cancer. The stage of a cancer is how doctors describe the extent of cancer in the body.[2] In the process of staging your cancer, your doctor is asking: how big is your tumor? Has the cancer spread to other parts of your body (metastasized)? How far has the cancer spread? What organs are involved? What is the topography of the cancer in your body?

For example, if we diagnose breast cancer, the questions doctors ask during staging are: what is the size of the primary tumor? Are we looking at a cancer that has spread to the axillary lymph nodes—the lymph nodes in the armpit? Has it spread to the lungs, liver, into a bone? Has the cancer advanced beyond the breast and, if so, how far? These are the questions answered by staging.

Staging your cancer is extremely important because every stage of cancer has a different treatment. You and your doctor need to know the stage of your cancer before you can discuss the best possible course of treatment.

~

The best way to assess the anatomic extent of a cancer is to conduct imaging studies. Many of the imaging studies we use to stage cancer have been in use for many years, and a number of new technologies and techniques have been developed recently. With these tools, doctors can determine more precisely than ever before just how far a cancer has spread.

The imaging studies we typically use to determine the stage of a cancer include computed tomography (CT) scan, magnetic resonance imaging (MRI), bone scan and positron emission tomography (PET) scan. Each of these different technologies has unique capabilities for the staging of cancer, but certain accommodations or precautions may be required for some patients. Before any studies are done, it is important to talk to your doctor about the benefits of these tests and any test-related accommodations and precautions you may require.

A CT scan is an X-ray picture of the body.[3] However, unlike the X-rays you may have had before, in which the X-ray machine takes a single quick picture from just one side of your body, the CT scanner rotates the X-ray beam all the way around your body, so that the pictures show your body in cross-section. During a CT scan, you lie on a table and the table is moved into the center of the CT scanning machine. This allows the X-ray beam to rotate all the way around you.

The CT scanning machine takes many, very thin, cross-section pictures in a series. Each picture is called a slice. When stacked together by the computer, the slices create a three-dimensional image of the part of the body that was scanned. These cross-sectional and three-dimensional images allow doctors to look all the way into and through your body.

CT scans may focus on specific parts of your body, or your doctor may order a full body CT scan. Sometimes contrast agents are given to patients to enhance the X-ray pictures taken. The advantage of a CT scan is that it provides doctors with a high-resolution image of your body which doctors can use to identify many different kinds of anatomic abnormalities, including cancerous tumors.

An MRI is a bit like a CT scan in that you lie on a table which is moved into the center of the MRI scanner, but, instead of using X-rays, an MRI machine uses a large magnet and radio waves to take pictures of your body.[4,5] Because MRI scanners use a different method for taking pictures, MRI scans provide doctors with different types of information than are obtained from CT scans. Like CT scans, MRI scans provide doctors with high-resolution images of your body which are used to identify a variety of abnormalities, including cancerous tumors. MRI scans may also require that contrast agents be given to patients to enhance the pictures taken, and MRI scans may focus on one or more parts of your body. Many patients complain that MRI machines make a lot of noise, and the inside of the machine is quite confining.

Bone scans and PET scans, sometimes called scintigraphy, are nuclear imaging tests that are performed and interpreted by specialists in nuclear medicine. During the tests, technicians will introduce very small amounts of a radioactive tracer material into your body, so that the imaging systems can evaluate the areas of your body in which the radioactive material accumulates.

In a bone scan, the radioactive material that is injected into your body is taken up by your bones.[6,7] The radiation emitted by the injected material is detected by a camera that moves around you while you lie on a table. A bone scan looks at how the radioactive tracer that is injected into your body is taken up by your bones. The scan can be used to identify a variety of abnormalities within your bones. The abnormalities are detected because they interrupt the way the radioactive tracer would normally be distributed within your bones. In cancer staging, a bone scan is used to determine whether cancer is present in the bone.

In a PET scan, the radioactive material is taken up by your organs and tissues.[8,9] Although PET scans do not show as much anatomic detail as a CT or MRI scan, they are exceptional for

Fiona's story

Fiona was diagnosed with breast cancer. Her doctors performed CT and MRI scans of her breasts, a bilateral mammogram, an ultrasound of the axillary lymph nodes and bone scans. With these studies, Fiona's doctors did not detect any evidence of cancer outside Fiona's breasts, so they performed a mastectomy—surgery to remove her breast. But Fiona did not receive a PET scan before surgery.

After surgery, a PET scan was performed, and Fiona's doctors found evidence of cancer in her liver.

Had Fiona gotten the PET scan before surgery, her mastectomy would have been contraindicated (advised against). This is because once breast cancer has spread to the liver, a mastectomy will not remove the cancer from the body. Fiona needed systemic treatment—chemotherapy that goes to the entire body—not surgery.

Because the staging of Fiona's cancer was not complete before her treatment was begun, Fiona underwent a surgical intervention that would not help her.

Gerald's story

Gerald came to see me after surgery for colon cancer. Before his surgery, Gerald's doctors ordered a CT scan of his liver. The CT scan was negative, so Gerald's doctors performed surgery on his colon.

However, colon cancer tends to spread to the liver. And the problem is that occasionally a liver CT will be negative when a PET scan would be positive. This is because a PET scan is a more sensitive test for cancer than a CT.

So, when Gerald came to see me, I did a total body PET scan which showed metastatic cancer in Gerald's liver.

Had Gerald's PET scan been performed prior to his surgery, his surgery would have been contraindicated (advised against). Based on the results of the PET scan, Gerald needed systemic chemotherapy, not surgery.

But, because staging of Gerald's cancer was incomplete at the time of his surgery, he faced the risks and consequences of a surgery that would not help him.

examining how your organs and tissues are working. Like an MRI, the patient lies on a table and the table is moved inside a scanner. PET scans can help diagnose a variety of medical conditions. For example, PET scans can check blood flow in the heart to investigate damage done by a heart attack, map functional abnormalities of the brain or determine the extent of cancer in the body. In most cases, a PET scan is the most important imaging study for staging cancer, because it is the most sensitive for detecting cancer in the body.

Today, many hospitals have instruments that are combined CT and PET scanners. When used in combination, these scans can give us highly detailed information on the extent of a disease like cancer. The CT scan determines the anatomy—it allows us to detect and localize a nodule or a suspicious mass. The PET scan distinguishes how that mass is functioning biochemically—it shows us the difference between a mass that is benign and a mass that is malignant based on the metabolism of the mass.

The specific technologies we need to use in order to stage a particular cancer differ from one type of cancer to another. Some or all of these methods may be needed to stage your cancer. Also, there may be other tests your doctor orders, depending on the type of cancer you have. For example, your doctor may use ultrasound imaging, which relies on high frequency sound waves, to examine your tumor. Your doctor may also use tumor markers to help stage your cancer.[10] As you will recall from Chapter 1, tumor markers are often used in the diagnosis of cancer, but tumor markers can also be used in staging a cancer. This is because, for some cancers, the levels of a particular tumor marker may serve as an indication of how advanced the cancer is.

It can be frustrating, inconvenient and uncomfortable to undergo a variety of different tests, and you may not always understand the need, but each test provides a unique view of your cancer. By ordering various tests, your doctor is simply trying to get the best information he or she can, based on the type of cancer you have, in order to stage your cancer as accurately as possible. It is important to do this so that you and your doctor can make the best decisions possible as you plan the next steps in your journey.

∼

Henry's story

Henry was a healthy man but a chronic smoker. He had a headache that would not go away. After a week, he went to his doctor. Henry's doctor performed blood tests, a chest X-ray and an EKG—a test that evaluates the heart's electrical activity, also called an electrocardiogram or ECG.

On the chest X-ray, Henry's doctor saw a lesion in Henry's right lung. Because Henry was a heavy smoker, his doctor was suspicious of this lesion and ordered a chest CT which showed that the suspicious lesion looked like primary lung cancer.

Henry's doctor referred Henry to a medical oncologist who performed a CT of Henry's chest, abdomen and pelvis, and bone scans. No evidence of cancer outside Henry's lung was found by these studies so Henry had surgery to remove his right lung.

About two weeks later, Henry came to see me because his headache was worse than ever.

Lung cancer frequently goes to the brain and Henry had a headache, so I did an MRI of Henry's brain which showed metastatic cancer.

Remember, Henry originally saw his doctor complaining of a headache but, after detecting Henry's lung cancer, his doctors did not pursue his original complaint—none of Henry's doctors ordered a brain MRI before his lung surgery. However, had Henry's doctors known prior to surgery that he had metastatic brain cancer, the surgery to remove his lung would have been contraindicated.

The point is: because an MRI of Henry's brain was not done prior to surgery, staging of Henry's cancer was not complete, and Henry had a surgery that would not help him.

It is also important to make sure that, in the process of staging your cancer, you and your doctor pay attention to all of your symptoms. Tell your doctor about the symptoms you have, even if you think some of them might not be related to your cancer. Some symptoms could indicate the spread of your cancer beyond the organ or tissue of origin; don't get so focused on your diagnosed cancer that you and your doctor overlook symptoms that might be connected to it. Take a step back, and make sure you and your doctor look at the big picture. You will have to help your doctor do this because only you can tell your doctor about all of your symptoms.

You might also have to keep reminding your doctor about all the symptoms you have. It may be difficult to imagine how some symptoms, especially common complaints such as headaches or low back pain might be related to your cancer. You might think they are just common problems that lots of people have—and you could be right. But these assumptions make some symptoms easy to ignore. If you have cancer, do not just assume that your symptoms could not possibly be related to your cancer. Remind your doctor about your symptoms, and investigate your symptoms with your doctor. Take the time to do the studies necessary to find out whether your symptoms are related to your cancer.

Unless your doctor can rule out a connection between a symptom and cancer, you cannot know for sure that the symptoms you have are not related to your cancer. Often, symptoms do turn out to be related to the cancer, so you have to investigate the relationship. For example, if a patient has a lung lesion and a headache, the first question should be whether it is related. If a patient has back pain and cancer, could the back pain be due to metastatic cancer in the bone? If any of the symptoms you have are related to your cancer, it could change your treatment.

Isaac's story

Isaac has prostate cancer, specifically prostate adeno-carcinoma.

In staging prostate cancer, we go by something called the Gleason score which is a measure of a tumor's malignancy, that is, how different the tumor is from normal prostate tissue. Gleason scores range 2-10. If a patient receives a Gleason score of 2-4, they will generally do well after treatment. Anything under a score of 5 is considered very favorable. But a Gleason score of 8-10 signifies a very malignant tumor. Usually prostate tumors with a Gleason score of 8-10 have already spread at the time of diagnosis.

Isaac's Gleason score was 10.

Isaac also had low back pain that was not too severe. Isaac's back was evaluated with a bone scan which was negative.

Isaac had a radical prostatectomy—surgery to remove his prostate. But the pain in his back continued to get worse.

The problem in Isaac's case is that a bone scan may not always detect cancer in the spine. A better test for the spine is an MRI. But an MRI of Isaac's lower back was not performed before his surgery.

When Isaac's back pain continued to worsen, an MRI of his lumbar spine was finally done, and it revealed that some vertebrae in his back were damaged by cancer.

Had Isaac's doctors performed the MRI of his spine before surgery, the stage of his cancer would have contraindicated the removal of his prostate, because the surgery could not have removed the cancer from Isaac's body. Instead, Isaac should have received systemic treatment and radiation.

Furthermore, cancer patients often get referred to other doctors in the course of their treatment—specialists who are experts in treating their type of cancer. Information sometimes gets lost when a patient is transferred from one doctor to another. A doctor may not see a potential relationship between a particular symptom and your cancer, so the symptom is not specifically brought to the attention of the new doctor during referral. For example, your doctor may not know that prostate cancer spreads preferentially to bone, or that colon cancer spreads preferentially to the liver. Your doctor may not be aware that lung cancer is notorious for spreading to the brain. So, when you are referred to a new doctor, such as a medical oncologist or other cancer specialist, make sure the information and records related to all the symptoms you have, even if they seem common and unlikely to be related to your cancer, make the transfer with you. Take the time to talk to your new doctor about all your symptoms, just to make sure they get attention.

In addition to talking about any symptoms you have when you first see your doctor, it is important that you and your doctor take the time to revisit your overall health status periodically. Make sure to talk to your doctor about any new symptoms you may experience as you develop them. It may seem an obvious thing to do, but such discussions often do not happen because they are time-consuming and can be rife with inaccuracies, imperfect memories and confounding factors.

So, bring up all of your symptoms, repeatedly if necessary, and reevaluate them from time to time. Make sure that you and your doctor are confident that you have ruled out an association between any symptoms you have and your cancer. The staging of your cancer is not complete until all of your symptoms have been addressed, and completing the staging of your cancer is necessary if you and your doctor are to make the best possible choices as you consider your treatment options.

~

Finally, it is important to remember that every cancer is different. The imaging and tests required for complete staging differ for different types of cancer and for different patients, and may depend on your symptoms. In some cases, the staging of a cancer might require quite extensive imaging studies. Unfortunately, extensive imaging is sometimes not done at the point of staging because imaging tests are time-consuming, expensive and may not be covered by third-party payors.

Advocate for yourself with your doctor and your payor. You may have to be persistent, but if you and your doctor think a test is important, talk about whether the test should be done, how it can be done, whether your payor will cover it and, if it will not, whether you or your doctor can appeal to the payor and assert the medical necessity of the testing—especially if the test is being ordered because of a particular symptom that you have. You or your doctor might be able to convince your payor to cover the cost of the test. There may also be other options for funding in your area such as charitable organizations, or you may decide to pay for some tests out of pocket if you and your doctor think they are important.

The point I am making is that this step in your journey, the step of staging your cancer, is very important. Staging is not complete until all the studies needed to stage your type of cancer are done, and staging needs to be complete if you and your doctor are to make the best decisions about your course of treatment.

~

Now that you have undergone all of the imaging studies and other tests required, the staging of your cancer is complete, and you know if, and how far, the cancer has spread in your body, let's move on to the next step in your journey: the group consultation.

3

THE GROUP CONSULTATION

When we collaborate... the whole is greater than the sum of its parts.

KEITH SAWYER, PH.D. [1]

Cancer poses complex challenges to both patients and physicians. For patients, the challenges involve the physical, psychological, social, financial and occupational implications of the diagnosis and of the, sometimes long term, complicated interventions needed to treat cancer. For physicians, cancer is unlike many other diseases because it is not often effectively managed by a single doctor with limited visits to the clinic or a single procedure or prescription.

Consider, for example, a medical diagnosis of the flu. The flu is often managed by one physician, perhaps a general practitioner or pediatrician. One or two limited-duration prescriptions may be written, and a patient may go to the doctor's office only once or twice before the virus has cleared and treatment is ended. More complicated is an underactive thyroid (called hypothyroidism). Hypothyroidism may be managed by an endocrinologist or perhaps a general practitioner, sometimes separately or perhaps jointly. One or more long-duration prescriptions may be required, and a patient may need to return to the doctor's office regularly for follow-ups and tests, but often no more than one or perhaps two doctors are needed for ongoing management.

In contrast, the treatment of cancer can be much more of a challenge. The treatment of cancer commonly requires a multi-disciplinary team consisting of many different cancer specialists, each with their own particular areas of skill and expertise. This is because cancer is a complex disease. If the cancer has not spread beyond the site of the primary tumor, the goal is to prevent its spread. To achieve this goal, some combination of surgery, radiation, chemotherapy, immunotherapy and other interventions may be employed. If the cancer has spread beyond the site of the primary tumor, a broader, more systemic approach to treatment may be required which often involves chemotherapy or immunotherapy.

The treatment of cancer may also require a long-term approach with multiple visits to various doctors over months or years. Such a complex course of treatment requires teamwork that takes into consideration not only a patient's immediate treatment needs, but also anticipates long-term treatment, surveillance and follow-up and, ultimately, contemplates the endgame: beating the cancer. This is why the treatment of cancer is frequently best designed by a group working together. Consequently, before I start therapy for any of my cancer patients, I like to obtain a group consultation.

This group consultation is the next step in your journey toward treatment of your cancer and many physicians will join your journey on this step.

~

In my group consultations, I bring all the specialists who will be involved in treating my patient together in a room at the same time. We review and discuss every aspect of the patient's medical status including the diagnosis, pathology findings, scans obtained from imaging studies, results of blood tests if any were done, and the patient's full set of symptoms and their overall clinical condition. The goal is to devise the best possible strategy for treating my patient and his or her cancer.

The group consultation facilitates communication between all the specialists who will be involved in my patient's care. You've heard the expression "two heads are better than one". Well, this is the basic principle behind the group consultation—to get all of the various specialists to discuss recommendations for treatment as a group, listen to each other's ideas and arrive at a consensus treatment plan.

The group consultation also protects the patient and doctors from bad decisions made in isolation or in the absence of key information. By assembling together, the doctors can share information far more effectively than they can with one-to-one conversations. The doctors can consider different treatment options together, communicate the rationale behind each of their individual viewpoints, share their own experience and expertise and discuss concerns about various treatment options in a coordinated manner. In this way, the care team is assured that any treatment decisions have taken into account as much of a patient's medical information and as much medical knowledge, and skill, as possible.

An additional, perhaps less obvious but no less relevant, reason for having a group consultation is that such meetings are educational. No doctor knows everything, and medical knowledge is constantly changing and advancing. It is impossible for any one doctor to keep up with every new study or advance in every area of medicine. By discussing a patient's treatment options in a group consultation, doctors learn from each other. I have never been in a group consultation where I did not learn something new.

∼

A radiologist, cancer surgeon and medical oncologist often comprise the core of a group consultation. The radiologist is the person who performed the scans during staging. The radiologist will tell the group about the topography of the disease in the patient's body, helping to pinpoint exactly where the disease is located and how widespread it may be. Of course, anyone can look at a set of scans and reports on a computer, but the importance of the radiologist's participation in the group consultation cannot be understated. With the radiologist there, all the members of the team have the opportunity to review all the scans and ask questions of the radiologist face-to-face. Without the radiologist present, the members of the team typically would not have the opportunity to talk directly to the radiologist, and valuable information might not be brought up for discussion.

The cancer surgeon is the person who will perform surgery, should surgery be recommended. The surgeon will describe the surgical approaches that can be used to remove the cancer from the patient's body and the benefits and limitations of the various approaches.

The medical oncologist is the person who will oversee the patient's care throughout their treatment. The medical oncologist will discuss the patient's symptoms and general state of health and perhaps describe chemotherapy or other relevant treatments.

Other specialists are added to this core group as needed for the patient's care. The type of cancer, the stage of the cancer and the symptoms a patient has will determine the precise mix of doctors needed in a group consultation, and this mix may differ from one group consultation to another, but the key element is the group consultation itself. To be effective, the group consultation needs all the members of the care team to be present and involved. If one member of the care team is missing, the circle is broken.

Jane's story

Jane had leiomyosarcoma, a tumor of smooth muscle cells. Smooth muscle cells are involuntary muscle cells—muscle cells over which the brain does not exert conscious control. Smooth muscle is found throughout the body, but one example of smooth muscle is the muscle that lines the digestive tract.

As the team reviewed all of Jane's clinical information and test results during her group consultation, Jane's surgeon raised concerns about whether surgery would benefit Jane. He believed she would be best treated with radiation and chemotherapy, but I disagreed. I believed Jane needed surgery followed by radiation and chemotherapy. I was concerned that, without surgery to remove Jane's primary tumor, the radiation and chemotherapy would not be as effective in treating her cancer as they would be with surgery.

After consideration of all of Jane's clinical information and test results, and discussion of all the options for Jane's treatment, the team ultimately concluded that surgery followed by radiation and chemotherapy was the best course of action for Jane.

Jane is alive and well more than ten years later.

Some cases of cancer may require the involvement of more than one expert in a particular specialty. For example, I am a medical oncologist. In setting up a group consultation, I might call upon two or three medical oncologists to participate, or I might call in more than one surgeon, or more than one radiation oncologist. This is because I like to hear different opinions before we decide on a treatment strategy.

I also like to include my patient in my group consultations. This is because I want my patient to understand how and why a particular treatment plan was decided upon. Having the patient present gives him or her the chance to hear all the information and every viewpoint directly from each of their doctors, all at the same time. It also facilitates the patient's ability to ask questions of their doctors and allows every member of the care team to hear, and respond to, the patient's questions and concerns.

Group consultations are not without their challenges, however. One of the biggest challenges with a group consultation is that it can be difficult to get everyone in a room together. But the group consultation approach is, I believe, in the end much more efficient than trying to share all of this information in one-to-one conversations. Also, when everyone is together, the conversation changes. With everyone listening to everyone else, questions and concerns are often brought forward that might never have been thought of if the group had not been in a room together. For these reasons, I always find value in the group consultation.

～

Every team needs a captain. In my group consultations, the medical oncologist is the captain of the team—the chair of the

Kevin's story

Kevin had pancreatic cancer.

The pancreas is a large gland located beneath the stomach. The pancreas secretes insulin and other substances involved in controlling blood sugar levels and metabolism as well as enzymes that aid the digestion of food. Kevin's cancer was in the head of the pancreas —the portion of the pancreas that is situated within the curve of the duodenum, the upper part of the small intestine that connects to the stomach.

Pancreatic cancer is very serious, particularly when it occurs in the head of the pancreas—the largest part of the pancreas. The operation to remove cancer from the head of the pancreas is called a Whipple procedure, named for Dr. Allen Whipple, the doctor who first performed the procedure in the 1930s. The Whipple procedure is a difficult operation because there are many blood vessels in and around the head of the pancreas.

Kevin's cancer required a Whipple procedure but when his surgeon started the operation, he discovered that Kevin's tumor was larger than the pre-operative imaging suggested. Kevin's surgeon was concerned because he saw a lymph node next to the pancreas that was positive for cancer which indicated that the disease had spread from the pancreas. At that time in history, doctors thought that if the disease had spread from the pancreas, surgery would not help. So, Kevin's surgeon wanted to stop the surgery.

But I was in the operating room that day, and I urged Kevin's surgeon to continue the surgery. As a medical oncologist, I knew there were new drugs available for treating pancreatic cancer. I felt Kevin's best chance for survival was for the surgeon to go ahead with the surgery.

After lengthy discussion, Kevin's surgeon performed the Whipple procedure which I followed with chemotherapy.

Kevin is alive and well today, more than fifteen years after his surgery, with no evidence of recurrent cancer.

meeting. This is because the medical oncologist is going to be the point person for the patient throughout the course of treatment.

Many different doctors may be involved in providing medical treatment to a cancer patient at different points during the course of care, but the medical oncologist is typically the one person in charge of implementing the overall strategy that was decided on during the group consultation. The medical oncologist will be the one member of the care team that the patient sees regularly as the treatment plan is implemented—the one person keeping an eye on the big picture.

As the patient moves through surgery, radiation therapy or chemotherapy, the medical oncologist is there, perhaps in person, perhaps on the phone, but continuously watching the patient's progress. If a problem arises, the medical oncologist can manage the problem or call the group together again to discuss the treatment plan and address whether modifications to the plan are needed. For my patients, I am always monitoring their care and progress. I have even found it important to be present in the operating room when decisions have to be made in real time based on unexpected circumstances.

Having a team captain is also important so that the patient knows he or she has one doctor in charge of coordinating all the various treatments—one doctor who is a main point of contact no matter where the patient may go or which other member of the care team they see. This is especially important in large or fragmented institutions—patients need to know they have someone they can rely on to take care of them.

I often explain it this way: the surgeon's responsibility is to perform a procedure to remove a cancer and to monitor the patient's post-operative recovery, and the radiation oncologist's responsibility is to perform the procedures to deliver radiation to a tumor in order to shrink the size of the tumor. But these may be time-limited events. A patient may see a surgeon or radiation oncologist for a defined period of time and then not again. Over a long course of treatment, the medical oncologist is always there.

∾

At the end of the group consultation, the care team should have a treatment strategy for the patient and be agreed on what steps will be taken and in what order. For example, the team may have decided that surgery will be done first, followed by radiation and then chemotherapy. The group consultation also provides an understanding of who will be responsible for which aspects of the patient's care.

Once determined, individual members of the care team will implement the treatment strategy based on their particular areas of expertise, while the medical oncologist keeps watch over the patient's progress. But initiation of treatment does not mean the group effort is over. It is important that the care team stay functional throughout a patient's entire course of treatment, so they can come together again, in person or by phone, for additional conversations when needed. It is not uncommon for there to be many group consultations throughout the course of a patient's treatment. To be optimally effective, the care team needs to be a dynamic group that remains engaged in the patient's care until treatment is completed.

∾

The unfortunate truth is that many cancer doctors do not do group consultations. There may be many reasons for this. It can be remarkably difficult to find a single time during which the entire team can assemble in a room together. Doctors' practices within large institutions or groups of affiliated institutions can become fragmented, so that one specialty or department has difficulty coordinating or communicating with another. The restrictions of insurance plans may lead to a patient seeing doctors from different, unaffiliated practice groups that may have difficulty sharing information. There may be an absence of certain specialties in a given location, and asking a doctor to leave his or her practice and travel from a remote location to join a group consultation may be impractical.

For these, and many other reasons, patients often go to see each of the various doctors on their care team sequentially and on their own. When this happens, a patient may get a different viewpoint from each of the different doctors about what interventions are needed and when—these viewpoints may even contradict one another. This can lead to confusion for the patient and uncertainty about what needs to be done next and why. This may also cause a patient to lose confidence in the medical team.

Additionally, when a patient sees various doctors individually, the doctors may not get the full clinical picture for the patient because they do not have the opportunity to talk directly to one another. Each individual doctor may not understand, or even know, the opinions of the other doctors who will take care of the patient. In contrast, the group consultation, while potentially challenging to coordinate, avoids these difficulties for both patients and doctors.

~

Often, cancer patients do not seek a second opinion. When they do, patients may seek these additional opinions on their own and without input from the doctors they have already seen. Perhaps the patient is concerned about offending a doctor if he or she finds out that the patient wants to talk to another physician. For the patient, however, such an approach can further fragment care and result in even more conflicting information and recommendations than they might have already received. And for doctors, such an approach can lead to confusion about who is going to take care of the various aspects of the patient's care and the overall treatment plan.

Instead, the group consultation, as I have described it, by its very nature, provides second opinions, and often third and fourth opinions—all at one time—and it allows all these views to be heard by everyone participating in the patient's care. And who better than the team captain to know just which doctors to call upon for those second and third opinions?

~

So, I urge you to seek treatment at a center with a multidisciplinary team approach to treating cancer. I recognize, however, that not all patients will live in places that have such resources available. If you do not live someplace where a multidisciplinary team is close by, or you are unable to access such resources for some other reason, you and your doctor may be able to form a team by telephone, telemedicine or other such means. Work with your doctor to use all the tools at your disposal to assemble a coordinated team and conduct your group consultation.

You may also be tempted to seek out information on the Internet. Many people do this, but do not confuse information found online with a second opinion or a group consultation. Medicine is multifaceted, cancer is complex and every patient is unique. Use caution when searching for and reading medical information online. Make sure that the resources you access are reliable, authoritative resources. Keep in mind that, since the information provided online by even the most reliable sources is usually generalized to large populations, it may not apply to you specifically or to your type or stage of cancer and may not be frequently updated. In fact, this is true for any medical information found online about any condition, not just cancer. Always talk to your doctors about any information you find, especially before taking any action based on that information.

Through the course of your treatment, you may also come into contact with other people who have, or have been treated for, a type of cancer similar to yours. Again, be careful about the information and recommendations they offer. This is true whether they are talking about cancer or another medical condition. It does not mean their suggestions and experience do not have value and were not correct for them at the time, but their experiences are their own and may not apply to you. Be sure to talk to your doctors before making any decisions or taking any action on the advice of individuals who are not your doctors.

∾

Now that you have had your group consultation, and you and your team of doctors have agreed upon the best possible strategy for treating your cancer, let's move on to the next step in your journey: preparing for treatment.

4

Preparing for Treatment

All things are ready if our minds be so.

WILLIAM SHAKESPEARE[1]

Now that your cancer has been diagnosed and staged, and your multidisciplinary care team has decided upon the best treatment plan for you, it is time to prepare for the start of your treatment. This may sound like a simple thing: you make a bunch of appointments and show up—the rest is up to your doctors. But, in fact, preparing for the start of your cancer treatment is not nearly so simple. There are many things to discuss.

When my patients reach this stage in their journey, I like to have them come to my office for a planning meeting. This meeting is different from the group consultation meeting. The group consultation was a strategic meeting—to establish a long-range plan, set goals and determine the means for achieving those goals. In contrast, the planning meeting is a tactical meeting—to lay out the actions, go over the details, set expectations and plan for contingencies. The purpose of it is to map out the logistics of treatment.

This planning meeting also involves different people to those present at the group consultation. Of course, a few of the people who participated in the group consultation may also be in the planning meeting, but there are other people at the planning meeting, people you may not have met yet, but who will join you at this step of your journey.

~

The main participant in the planning meeting is the patient. The primary purpose of the planning meeting is to talk about what is to come.

In my experience, patients who are preparing to start treatment for cancer tend to have many detailed and specific questions. They are anxious and want to know what to expect. The planning meeting is the time to answer these questions.

~

One of the first things I do in my planning meetings is go over specific actions and activities involved in the treatment plan. We talk about the major steps of the treatment plan and discuss the big issues involved. Such a discussion often leads us rapidly into the details.

If surgery is planned, I find that my patients want to know how soon the surgery can be scheduled. They often ask:

- What will the operation itself be like?
- What tests and procedures will have to be performed before surgery?
- What will my pre-op instructions be?
- Will I have to stay in the hospital? If so, how long will I have to stay in the hospital?
- How painful will the surgery be?

- What medications can I expect to be given before, during or after surgery?
- How long will I have to take these medications?
- How do I take these medications?
- Will these medications interact with other medications I take?
- What will the post-operative recovery process be like?
- What tests and procedures will need to be performed after surgery?
- Will I need home care after I leave the hospital?
- What will I be able to do when I go home?
- What can I not do when I go home?
- Will I need physical therapy or rehabilitative care after surgery?
- How long will it be before I can return to normal activities?
- When can I expect to return to work?

If radiation therapy or chemotherapy is planned, I find my patients want to know when the treatments will begin. They often ask:

- What will the treatments themselves be like?
- Will they be painful? Will they make me feel bad?
- Will my hair fall out?
- Will I have to do anything before treatment to prepare?
- How long will each treatment session take?
- How many sessions will there be?
- Over what period of time will the sessions occur?
- Will I have to stay in the hospital before or after the treatment sessions? If so, for how long?

- Are there side effects related to the treatments?
- How will my care team help me handle any side effects I have from treatment?
- How long after treatment will it take for me to feel better?
- What other medications can I expect to be given before, during or after treatment?
- How long will I have to take these medications?
- How do I take these medications?
- Will these medications interact with other medications I take?
- Will my activities be restricted as a result of treatment?
- Will I have specific instructions to follow after treatment?
- Will I need help taking care of myself or my family as a result of the treatments?
- How long will it be before I can return to normal activities?
- How much time will I have to take off work because of the treatments?

My patients also want to know what their calendar is going to look like. They often ask:

- How will the various treatments disrupt daily life?
- What about other plans such as family activities, parties, graduations, weddings, holidays and vacation or travel plans?

If my patients are traveling to receive care, they often ask:

- How long will I be at the care facility? Can I drive there, or do I need to fly?

- Will I need a car once I get to the treatment facility?
- Where can I stay that is conveniently located for getting to the hospital or treatment facility?
- How many trips will I have to make to complete my treatment?
- What will I need to do about food, medicines and other necessities while traveling?
- Can I bring a family member or friend with me for my treatments? Who might be best?
- What impact is being with me going to have on their activities and responsibilities?

My patients also want to know about post-treatment follow-up appointments and tests. They often ask:

- How many follow-up appointments will I have?
- What will these follow-up appointments be like?
- How much time will they take?
- How often will they occur and over what time period?
- What follow-up tests or procedures will I need to have?
- How often will I need to have these tests or procedures?
- How might the results of these tests or procedures change my treatment plan?
- Will I be placed on any long-term medications?
- How do I take these medications?
- What are the side effects of these medications?
- Will these medications interact with other medications that I take?

Depending upon how involved your treatment plan is, and how many questions and concerns you have, planning meetings can take quite a lot of time. More than one planning meeting may be necessary, and it is always reasonable to expect that new questions or concerns will arise over the course of your treatment.

～

I also encourage my patients to bring their family with them to the planning meeting, along with anyone else they want to involve. These people are often afraid and uncertain about what to expect. They, too, may have many questions about what is to come and how it will impact their loved one and themselves.

This is very important. These people will support and care for my patient throughout his or her treatment. By inviting family and others to the planning meeting, my patients and their caregivers are all able to learn together about the next steps. Caregivers also get to meet the team that will be taking care of their loved one, collect contact information in case of emergency and be informed about how the care team will respond to unexpected problems should they arise.

～

Another group for whom the planning meeting is very important is my staff. The planning meeting may be the first opportunity some of my staff have to meet the patient.

At my practice in the Texas Medical Center, I am fortunate to work with a group of talented and compassionate professionals who are as devoted to my patients as I am. One of these incredible professionals is our nurse specialist and clinical administrator. I have had a few nurse specialists in my practice over the years, so, for the purpose of this chapter, I'll collectively call them all Linda.

Linda is a tremendous asset to my patients and to me. She is a source of information and support and she works closely with my patients to make sure they are completely ready for the journey they are about to take with their treatment. Linda is also available to my patients twenty-four hours a day, seven days a week throughout the course of their treatment.

My patients ask Linda many questions. They might even ask Linda the same questions that they have asked me. I do not mind this. I do not believe my patients mistrust me. They are faced with cancer and are about to begin a long fight against their disease. They only wish to be reassured, to be certain that the decisions they are making in their fight against cancer are the right ones.

I also include the staff from my business office in the planning meeting. I find that patients generally have many questions about the cost of treatment, how they will pay for it and what aspects of care their insurance might cover, be it health, supplemental, disability or long-term care insurance.

My business office staff have a great deal of experience with the financial side of treatment, and they capably go over the costs of treatment with the patient and the patient's family. My staff can also help the patient and family anticipate when bills will come and when payment will be due, and they can talk to patients about payment options and financial planning.

The role of supportive therapy is also an important topic for planning meetings. One type of supportive therapy we discuss in planning meetings is medical supportive therapy. Medical supportive therapy is treatment given daily, or on some other schedule, to control the complications of cancer and cancer treatment and make my patient's quality of life as normal as possible throughout the course of treatment. Medical supportive therapy can include intravenous (IV) fluids, IV medications, injected medications and/ or oral medications. For example, chemotherapy drugs often have the side effect of reducing a patient's white or red blood cell counts. If a patient's white blood cell count goes down, the patient becomes more susceptible to infection. If a patient's red blood cell count drops, the patient becomes anemic and may feel tired. Medical supportive therapy can deliver medications to boost white or red blood cell counts and counteract these effects of treatment.

My staff and I also help our patients understand and consider the value of psychological and social supportive therapy to help with all that they are going through. Depending on the type and stage of cancer, the patient's psychological well-being and the social environment surrounding the patient, supportive therapy may include psychological counseling, social and interpersonal guidance, and behavioral or physical therapies. Supportive therapies can also include helping patients and their family members adjust and adapt to new lifestyle patterns and to deal with limitations in activities which the patient may not have previously had.

～

Finally, I talk to my patients about their legal rights. We talk about the right to privacy, wills, directives to physicians and powers of attorney. We talk about the right to choose to stop treatment at any time, and we talk about what stopping treatment might mean, should the patient choose to do so at some point.

∾

At the conclusion of the planning meeting, the entire journey has been mapped out and our patients and their families are better informed about the treatments planned. This is the time when hope and optimism are very important. This is all likely to be new to patients, and new experiences can be worrying and overwhelming. But once my patients know they are in the hands of people who have done this for years, they feel reassured. And when my patients come to our office for chemotherapy or a visit with our doctors, we make sure they feel at home.

By taking some of the uncertainty out of what is to come, and giving our patients the support and reassurance they need in a place they feel comfortable, we strive to make this difficult journey a little bit easier. My patients often tell me that, as a result of the planning meeting, they realize that they are not alone—that we are walking with them every step of the way.

∾

Unfortunately, not all doctors hold planning meetings with their patients. There are many reasons your doctor may not set up a planning meeting. Time is often a major barrier to meetings such as this. Also, your doctor may not have the staff resources to hold such meetings. However, if your doctor does not offer to set up a planning meeting, I urge you to ask for one. If your doctor is unable to accommodate your request, then ask your doctor to connect you to the patient services departments at the institutions where you will be receiving your treatments. You may have to advocate for yourself a bit, but do not give up. Make sure you do everything you need to in order to be as prepared as possible for the start of your treatment.

∾

Now that you have had your planning meeting and are prepared for your treatment, let's move on to the next step in your journey: treating your cancer.

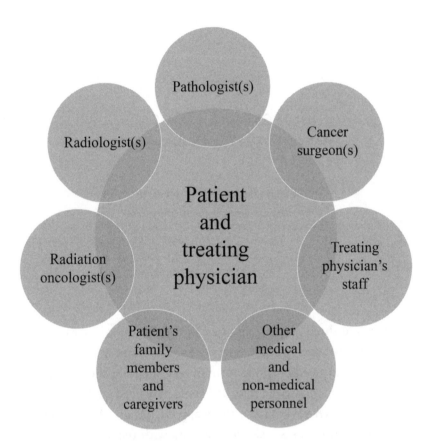

FIGURE 1 Diagram illustrating the centrality of the patient and treating physician in the treatment of cancer and the interconnectedness of the cancer care team. The patient and treating physician are always at the center of the diagnosis and treatment of the patient. Depending on the type and stage of a patient's cancer, other members are included in the team, but all remain connected to the patient and treating physician throughout the course of treatment.

5

SURGERY: A MEDICAL ONCOLOGIST'S PERSPECTIVE

To attain the best possible results the
physician and surgeon must co-operate.

SIR WILLIAM OSLER, M.D.
AND THOMAS MCCRAE, M.B. (TOR.)[1]

There are three approaches used in the treatment of cancer: surgery, radiation therapy and systemic therapy. Some cancer patients may need only one form of treatment for their cancer, some patients may need two, and some may need all three. The order in which we combine these approaches may be different for different patients, even for patients with the same type of cancer.

For some patients, the treatment of cancer begins with surgery. Selecting your cancer surgeon is an important step in the start of your cancer treatment. This is because not every surgeon is a cancer surgeon. Many surgeons are general surgeons. General surgeons are trained to perform a variety of different types of operations, and they are highly qualified to do so, but they are not cancer surgeons. Some surgeons are specialized. For example, orthopedic surgeons or heart surgeons are highly skilled in their areas of expertise, but they may not be trained in cancer surgery.

Cancer surgeons are different. Cancer surgeons have particular knowledge, skills and experience that help them understand the clinical context of cancer and what to look for when they are performing an operation on a patient with cancer. Cancer surgeons have awareness of the other types of treatments cancer patients may undergo and how those treatments might be impacted by the choices made during surgery. Cancer surgeons are also experts in the—sometimes complex and delicate—surgical techniques required to remove cancer from the body while preserving as much of the structure and function of surrounding tissues as possible.

But the specialization of cancer surgeons does not end simply with being a cancer surgeon—not all cancer surgeons can do every type of cancer surgery. Cancer is so complex that cancer surgeons often subspecialize. This means that there are cancer surgeons specifically trained in the operative techniques required to treat head and neck cancer or brain cancer or prostate cancer, and so on. For many cancer patients, a subspecialized cancer surgeon may be the best option. As the captain of your team, your medical oncologist can help you identify the best cancer surgeon for your type of cancer.

One often has to look to large institutions or dedicated cancer centers to find subspecialized cancer surgeons. Unlike hypertension or diabetes, both of which can be treated in just about any clinical setting and with limited specialized equipment, cancer surgery frequently demands a highly sophisticated treatment environment. This is because cancer surgery may require unique instruments, specifically designed clinical, laboratory and operative facilities as well as specially trained personnel. These elements can be difficult to assemble without the financial and physical resources, and patient load, of a large institution or specialized care center. If you do not live near one of these centers, you may have to travel for your cancer surgery.

~

As the captain of my patient's care team, my role does not pause when my patient goes to surgery. I do not leave the surgeon to work alone. I work with the surgeon, often by being present in the operating room during surgery. I do this because I believe surgery is such an important step for cancer patients that it is best performed in co-operation, not isolation.

You may recall that we discussed in Chapter 3 how important it is for the treating physician, usually the medical oncologist, to be involved in every aspect of a cancer patient's care. I told you Kevin's story, about how I was in the operating room for Kevin's surgery when the surgeon encountered something unexpected as he began Kevin's operation. I explained how beneficial it was for me to be present in the operating room to discuss the unexpected findings, in real time, with Kevin's surgeon.

Kevin's case is not unique. In the operating room, there is always decision-making that occurs. I find it is often important for me, as the treating physician, to be in the operating room and see what the surgeon sees as the surgeon sees it. My being there gives the surgeon the opportunity to discuss any unexpected findings with me and consider the impact of those findings on the patient's overall treatment plan. In some cases, these discussions lead us to proceed with a surgery despite unexpected circumstances; in other cases, we might decide to stop a surgery. Regardless, by discussing the decision together, the surgeon and I know we will arrive at the best decision possible.

Laura's story

Laura had breast cancer. Her imaging tests suggested that her tumor was small, so her team decided a mastectomy was the best way to begin Laura's treatment. In the operating room, the first thing the surgeon did was to identify the sentinel lymph nodes for Laura's tumor.

Sentinel lymph nodes are the first lymph nodes through which a tumor drains.[2] Sentinel lymph nodes are identified in the operating room by injecting a tracer such as a dye near the tumor. The tracer drains from the area just as the tumor drains, and the sentinel lymph nodes pick up the color of the dye.

The rationale for identifying and testing the sentinel lymph nodes for cancer cells is this: for many types of cancer, when cancer cells leave the original tumor site to travel to other parts of the body, they follow the path by which the tumor drains, through lymph nodes. By looking for cancer cells in the sentinel lymph nodes, doctors can assess the likelihood that the cancer has spread beyond the original tumor site. If the sentinel lymph nodes are negative, it is possible the cancer has not spread. If the sentinel lymph nodes are positive, it is presumed the cancer has spread beyond the original tumor site—how far it has spread cannot be determined by testing sentinel lymph nodes, only that it has spread.

Laura's sentinel lymph nodes were positive for cancer cells, so the surgeon and I determined that it was best to stop her surgery. Laura would need chemotherapy—systemic treatment that attacks cancer throughout the body.

Try as I might, however, I cannot always be in the operating room with my patients during surgery. But as the captain of the team, I always insist that the surgeon communicate with me during surgery. I do not tell the surgeon how to operate, but I do insist that any unexpected findings are discussed with me and that any unanticipated decisions are made collaboratively, especially if the unexpected findings change the surgeon's original operative plan.

If you have to travel to a cancer center for your cancer surgery, it may be impossible for your treating physician or medical oncologist to be with you in the operating room. But many large institutions and specialized care centers today have technological resources that allow doctors in other locations to talk with a surgeon in the operating room or view a surgery over a secure Internet connection. If you have to travel to receive your surgery, talk to your doctor about how he or she might be able to remain in close contact during the operation.

∾

One final thought about cancer surgery is this: some cancers, such as small melanomas, or some lung, colon or thyroid cancers, can be cured by surgery, especially if they are caught early. When cancers are caught early, surgery offers a chance to remove the tumor from the body before the cancer can spread.

Early-stage cancers are sometimes caught during regular checkups. So I urge you to get regular checkups with your doctor. And if you have been found once to have an early-stage cancer, keep up with your regular checkups after your cancer is treated—even if your doctors tell you that you are cured. This is because cancer does sometimes recur. And if cancer does reappear, it remains important to treat the new cancer while it is still in its early stages.

Mark's story

Mark had colon cancer. Staging studies did not show any signs of cancer outside Mark's colon, so surgery was scheduled to remove his tumor.

But when we got Mark into the operating room, and the surgeon looked at Mark's liver, he saw what looked like a small cancer on the surface of the liver. The surgeon performed a biopsy of what we saw, and that biopsy confirmed our suspicion of cancer. We discussed this finding and made the decision to stop Mark's surgery and begin chemotherapy.

Six months later, we took Mark back to the operating room to remove the original tumor from his colon.

∾

Now that you've read my perspectives on cancer surgery, let's move on to talk about radiation therapy.

6

Radiation Therapy: A Medical Oncologist's Perspective

In the past, radiation treatment planning has been a very lengthy procedure. Now, with the aid of CT therapy-planning computer programs, we can position the therapy beams automatically with precision in a few minutes.

SIR GODFREY N. HOUNSFIELD[1]

Radiation therapy is often used to treat cancer. It is performed by radiation oncologists and radiotherapists. Radiation oncologists are physicians trained in the use of radiation to treat cancer. Radiotherapists are trained in the administration of radiation treatments to patients.

Radiation therapy works because the high-energy particles emitted from radioactive sources damage DNA. The purpose of radiation therapy is to inhibit cell division and accelerate cell death in treated cells. The goal of radiation therapy is to shrink tumors while minimizing the side effects of treatment by causing as little injury as possible to non-cancerous tissue.

Forty years ago, radiation therapy as we know it today did not exist. The discovery of atomic energy and how to harness its power, combined with advances in biomedical science and computer technology, have made radiation therapy a reality and led to the creation of sophisticated machines that generate high-intensity beams of radiation that can be precisely controlled.

Compared to surgery, radiation is a long-term treatment. In many cases, radiation therapy will take place after surgery, if surgery is required. Radiation therapy may take place before or after chemotherapy.

$\sim$

Depending upon the type of tumor, and its location, radiation therapy uses different methods to deliver radiation to the body.[2] One approach to radiation therapy, sometimes called external radiation therapy or external beam radiation therapy, uses high-technology machines to direct a narrow beam of radiation straight into a tumor. These machines target the exact location in the body where the radiation beam will go, regulate how much radiation will be delivered and adjust how wide the beam of radiation will be. External radiation therapy is usually given every day for a period of two to eight weeks.

Radiation therapy can also be delivered to cancer patients by the placement of radioactive material inside a patient's body, in or near the tumor. In this form of radiation therapy, sometimes called internal radiation therapy or brachytherapy, the radioactive material remains in the body for an extended period of time, constantly emitting high-energy particles that damage and kill cancer cells. Unlike the external delivery of radiation by a machine, this type of radiation therapy delivers a continuous dose of radiation to the tumor, instead of the limited dose that can only be delivered when a patient is in a machine.

External beam radiation therapy and brachytherapy are localized approaches to radiation therapy and they are the most common ways by which radiation therapy is delivered to patients. Some patients may receive both kinds of radiation therapy as part of their cancer treatment.

There is also a third type of radiation therapy that may be used in some patients. This type of radiation therapy, sometimes called systemic radiation therapy, involves the administration, to the entire body, of a radioactive compound that is designed to be taken up only by cancer cells. For example, the treatment of thyroid cancer may include systemic administration of a radioactive form of iodine called I-131. This therapy works because iodine is only taken up by thyroid cells. As a result, I-131 targets cancerous thyroid cells that may have escaped the original tumor site and destroys these cells. There are other examples of the systemic use of radiation therapy, but, because systemic radiation therapy requires a way to target the radiation directly to a particular type of cell, systemic radiation therapy is not an option for many cancers.

~

Side effects are a common challenge when using radiation therapy.[2] Despite our best efforts to minimize the effects of radiation therapy on surrounding tissues, the radiation will sometimes cause damage to tissue outside the tumor.

Side effects from radiation therapy vary from patient to patient. The chances of having side effects from radiation therapy depend upon the type of radiation treatment being used and the part of the body that is targeted.

Fatigue is the most common side effect of radiation therapy. Patients may not feel up to going to work or doing everyday activities. However, fatigue is usually temporary and will typically go away when the treatment is over.

Most patients receiving external radiation therapy will experience changes in the skin near the site where the radiation was administered. The skin may become dry and may itch or peel. This happens because healthy skin cells are damaged when the radiation beam passes through the skin on its way to the tumor.

Hair loss is not common with radiation therapy unless the treatment is given to the head for a brain tumor. Nausea and vomiting are also infrequent in radiation therapy unless treatment is delivered to the abdomen, but, if nausea and vomiting do occur, they are usually manageable.

Other side effects can also occur. For example, if treatment is delivered to the lung, patients may develop a cough; if treatment is delivered to the prostate, patients may develop a burning sensation during urination or erectile dysfunction.

～

An additional consequence of radiation therapy that we have begun to see in patients in recent years is the occurrence of a secondary tumor that may develop many years after radiation therapy has concluded. In the past we did not see this because patients did not live long enough after treatment for secondary tumors to develop. Today, however, with more effective treatments for cancer, patients may survive ten to fifteen years after initial treatment. These patients may return with a new tumor which has developed in the area where the radiation therapy was given. This type of cancer is not a recurrence of the original tumor; it is a new tumor that has developed because of the DNA damage caused by radiation exposure during radiation therapy. It is uncommon, however, for tumors that develop as a result of radiation therapy to be serious.

~

The chance of side effects and secondary tumors must be considered when radiation therapy is integrated into a patient's treatment plan. Physicians are always weighing up the question of harm versus benefit. This is sometimes called the risk-benefit ratio. It is something patients must also consider in consultation with their doctors. If you have concerns about the risks of various treatments for your cancer, talk to your doctors and find out what the risks and benefits are so that you can make an informed choice about your treatment. In most cases, the benefits of radiation therapy for cancer far outweigh the risks, but the risks and benefits should be discussed, and decisions should be made with a full understanding of the potential harms and likely advantages.

~

I do not usually go with my patients to radiation therapy. Unlike surgery, where the surgeon might encounter some unexpected circumstance that needs my input in the middle of surgery, the radiotherapist rarely needs input from me during the administration of treatment to my patient. The radiation oncologist generally just works within the treatment plan.

This is not to say that problems or unexpected circumstances do not occur during radiation therapy. They can and do, but the problems that occur during radiation therapy are different from the problems that can occur during surgery and, in my experience, usually do not require decision-making on the spot.

Even though I am not usually in the treatment room with my patients when they receive their radiation therapy, I still do not leave my patients to navigate radiation therapy on their own. I stay in contact with the radiation oncologist, so that I know how the treatments are proceeding and how my patient's tumor is responding. In my experience, the problems that can occur during radiation therapy are best managed collaboratively, with the radiation oncologist and the captain of the care team working together. Just as the surgeon and I work as a team, I work together with the radiation oncologist to address any problems or unexpected circumstances that may arise in the course of my patient's radiation therapy.

I also stay in touch with my patients throughout their radiation therapy treatments to keep updated on their progress, understand how they are feeling and treat side effects that occur. My patients who receive radiation therapy come to our clinic frequently to be monitored and receive medical supportive therapy if needed. You may recall we talked a bit about medical supportive therapy in Chapter 4. We will talk more about it in Chapter 9, but for now it is one of the things I address with my patients receiving radiation therapy.

∼

For some cancers, radiation therapy may be the only treatment needed, but this is rare. It is far more common for radiation therapy to be used in addition to surgery or systemic therapy. This is because, just like surgery, radiation therapy is usually local, which means it affects cancer cells only in the area being treated. But cancer is often not localized. Even if physicians cannot see evidence of cancer elsewhere in the body, it is possible that it does exist in another part of the body. For this reason, most patients who receive surgery or radiation therapy also receive a systemic treatment—treatment that is delivered to the entire body—such as chemotherapy or immunotherapy.

~

Now that you've read my perspectives on radiation therapy, let's hear the perspective of a radiation oncologist, Dr. Bin Teh. Then, we will discuss systemic therapy.

7

RADIATION THERAPY: A RADIATION
ONCOLOGIST'S PERSPECTIVE

Radiotherapy, in addition to surgery and systemic therapy, plays a very
important role in the management of cancer. With advances in computing
and technology, radiotherapy or the healing rays have become more precise
and "gentler" leading to improved cure rates and fewer side effects.

BIN S. TEH, M.D., F.A.C.R

Note to readers: This chapter was contributed by Bin S. Teh, M.D.,
F.A.C.R. I have worked with Dr. Teh for many years and referred
many of my patients to him for treatment. I asked Dr. Teh to write
this chapter because he is a specialist in the field of radiation therapy. The chapter is more technical than the preceding chapter on
radiation therapy, but I believe you will find Dr. Teh's perspectives
helpful as you navigate your journey with cancer.

~

Among the noteworthy success stories in modern cancer care
is the multidisciplinary approach. Working as a team has the
advantage of bringing all the important expertise together to
produce the best possible outcome and greatest chance of a cure

for the cancer patient. As you may recall from Chapter 3, often this team approach to cancer care includes a medical oncologist, surgeon, radiation oncologist, pathologist and diagnostic radiologist. Usually, the team is led by the medical oncologist.

As described in the previous chapter by Dr. Salem, radiotherapy plays a very important role in cancer management. In this chapter, I am going to present various aspects of radiation therapy from a radiation oncologist's perspective.

∾

I am honored and fortunate to work with Dr. Salem, who is a master and who believes that cancer patients are best managed by a team of experts. We consult and examine the patient at the first consultation together. We review the patient's imaging and pathology. We take into consideration the correct diagnosis, extent of disease and previous treatments as well as the patient's body and performance status, including other medical conditions and the patient's wishes. Then, we formulate a treatment plan that we believe offers the best chance for a cure, but not at the expense of side effects for the patient.

∾

Radiotherapy is an effective and proven standard of care treatment for cancer. Dr. Salem has described in the previous chapter the mechanism of action by which radiotherapy kills cancer cells, so I will not spend time on that here. I will remind you, however, that, unlike surgery, which is usually performed only once, radiotherapy is typically delivered daily, over a few minutes, for a few weeks. This is known as fractionated radiotherapy.

Fractionated radiotherapy obeys the principles of classical radiobiology, known as The Four R's. The first two R's stand for reassortment/redistribution and reoxygenation. These two R's describe the advantages of using fractionated radiotherapy to kill cancer cells. The fractioned treatment regimen allows more cancer cells to enter a sensitive phase of the cell cycle over the course of treatment and permits a reduction in the number of resistant, oxygen-deficient cancer cells, thus increasing the number of cancer cells destroyed by the treatment. The other two R's stand for repair and repopulation. These two R's describe the advantages fractionated radiotherapy offers to normal cells near the treatment area. For these two R's, spreading treatment over many days allows normal cells time to repair any damage caused by the treatment and repopulate, thus leading to less toxicity and improving the patient's tolerance of the radiotherapy.

Radiotherapy is used to treat both cancerous tumors and non-cancerous tumors such as meningioma, acoustic neuroma, pituitary adenoma and many others. The radiation dosage used for treatment depends on the tumor types and locations, whether the patient has received prior radiotherapy, the intent of treatment and whether the patient is getting concurrent systemic therapy.

When radiotherapy is used to treat cancer, one thing we have to decide is whether our treatment is intended to cure, palliate (reduce symptoms) or both. Once the intent is clearly stated to the patient, the patient's expectations are more realistic. Typically, when radiotherapy is used for a cure, the dosage is higher, and the fractionation regimen is longer—in the range of six to eight weeks.

Although, as oncologists, we always want to cure patients, I personally find palliative radiotherapy can also be very rewarding. For example, when a patient with metastatic cancer involving multiple bones has a lot of pain, he or she may need to take high doses of pain medication. These medications can cause a variety of side effects such as nausea, constipation and drowsiness. These side effects can profoundly affect the patient's quality of life. A short course of palliative radiotherapy over one to ten treatments can help with significant pain relief, eliminating the need for pain medications. I find this a truly rewarding experience, because it helps patients so much.

≈

Historically, radiation treatment has been viewed by many people, including certain non-oncologists, as only a palliative treatment with significant side effects which can negatively impact a patient's quality of life. However, in the modern era of radiation oncology, this fear among cancer patients and physicians alike needs to be dispelled.

I talk to my patients about the many advances in radiotherapy that have improved its capacity to cure cancer and reduce the occurrence of side effects. For example, the healing beams are now "gentler" and also more focused and precise. In addition, advances in treatment planning and delivery have made radiotherapy safer and permitted the delivery of higher radiation doses. Some examples of the new forms of external beam radiotherapy that have resulted from advances in radiotherapy include: three-dimensional conformal radiotherapy (3DCRT), intensity-modulated radiation therapy (IMRT), image-guided radiation therapy (IGRT), stereotactic radiosurgery (SRS) and stereotactic body radiotherapy (SBRT).[1-3]

When drawing up a treatment plan for a patient, the choice of which form of radiotherapy to use depends upon many factors, including the type, location and characteristics of a patient's cancer, and the capabilities and limitations of the various technologies.

∾

As you may recall from previous chapters, radiotherapy is a local treatment, like surgery. But, unlike surgery, radiotherapy is non-invasive and can be delivered in outpatient settings. Additionally, because of advances in computing and technology, today's radio-therapy treatments are generally well-tolerated by patients, including patients who cannot be operated on because of comorbidities (additional medical conditions), such as heart failure, which make surgery risky. For example, SBRT is now the treatment of choice for medically inoperable patients with early-stage lung cancers or oligo-metastatic (the limited spread of a few) lesions. There is also emerging data that supports non-invasive SBRT, even for medically operable patients with early-stage lung cancer. In fact, SBRT has been described as one of the most significant advances in radiation oncology over the last fifty years.

The successful clinical implementation of SBRT is the result of a modern radiotherapy machine called a linear accelerator. Linear accelerators have a number of sophisticated capabilities including image-based guidance to map and track tumors within the body, to adjust for movement of the tumor during breathing or other bodily functions and to precisely deliver high-energy radiation directly to the tumor. These capabilities permit a shorter course of treatment (up to five fractions), with a higher dose per fraction.[1-3]

∾

When working closely with a medical oncologist like Dr. Salem, I am confident that we can achieve not only the best treatment plan from the outset, but also better monitor and manage the progress and side effects of treatment, especially if the patient is getting chemotherapy and radiotherapy at the same time or chemotherapy before radiotherapy. For example, when a patient gets concurrent chemotherapy and radiotherapy for cancer, especially head and neck cancer, lung cancer or gastrointestinal or pancreatic cancer, side effects, such as swallowing problems, tend to occur slightly more frequently and be more severe. If side effects occur, I report them to Dr. Salem and he provides the patient with medical supportive therapy (i.e. nutritional support, hydration and medications) to help ease the symptoms. Through the team approach and joint efforts, the patient will generally tolerate combined treatments well and sail through to complete the treatment regimen without any interruption of treatment days. This approach helps improve the patient's quality of life.

∽

Another important advancement in cancer care is cancer immunotherapy. Today, we have a new generation of immunotherapy agents which target specific proteins on immune and cancer cells such as CTLA-4, PD-1 and PD-L1. Normally, these proteins function as checkpoints, and they help keep the immune system under control. But the immunotherapy agents that target these proteins remove the restraints from the immune system, activating T-cells to attack cancer cells.[4]

Combining immunotherapy and radiotherapy can have a greater effect on cancer and enhance the killing of cancer cells. The most exciting result with this combined approach is known as the abscopal effect, whereby the treatment response is seen in metastatic lesions outside the irradiated area. The simple explanation for the abscopal effect is that when cells die as a result of radiotherapy, tumor-associated antigens are produced, and these can in turn stimulate the local immune system. When this occurs, irradiated cancer cells die, and the activated T-cells travel to other parts of the body to kill cancer cells outside the irradiated areas.

The abscopal effect is more commonplace in recent years because technologies such as SBRT, which delivers a higher dose of focused radiation per fraction, are more commonly used and because radiotherapy is now more frequently used in conjunction with immunotherapy. Again, this example highlights the importance of a radiation oncologist working closely alongside a medical oncologist, as Dr. Salem and I do, because we have to both be aware of, and closely monitor, the side effects of the combined treatment approach.

∾

In closing, radiotherapy in the modern era is more precise and can be delivered more accurately than ever before. Today, we can administer highly focused radiation, or gentle healing rays, more safely to achieve better cure rates and reduced treatment-related toxicity and side effects. We can also now combine radiotherapy safely with surgery or systemic therapies, such as chemotherapy, hormonal therapy or immunotherapy, to better control cancer both locally and systemically. The important point here is that your cancer treatment team needs to work very closely together to achieve the important goal of a cancer cure without significant side effects.

8

SYSTEMIC THERAPY

The disease you see is often not all the disease there is.

PHILIP A. SALEM, M.D.

We have reached that point in your journey where we need to discuss the most traveled path in cancer treatment: systemic therapy. Systemic therapy is different from surgery and radiation therapy because, with the exception of systemic radiation therapy, surgery and radiation therapy only treat cancer in the part of the body that is operated on or irradiated. In contrast, systemic therapy attacks cancer throughout the body.

Cancer patients often need systemic therapy because cancer is usually a systemic disease. You might think of a tumor as a site-specific problem, but cancer cells multiply, and tumors grow. As a result, cancer cells can separate from the original tumor and travel to other parts of the body to form new tumors. We call this metastasis or metastatic disease, and this is what makes cancer a systemic disease.

You may remember we talked in Chapter 2 about staging cancer. We stage cancer to investigate whether a patient has metastatic disease. Often, metastatic disease can be seen through the use of imaging technologies. You may also recall that in Chapter 5 we discussed how surgeons can test sentinel lymph nodes during cancer surgeries. This is another good way to investigate whether a tumor has metastasized. Staging studies are important because their results provide valuable information that guide decisions about the best treatment plan for a cancer patient. For example, if the staging studies indicate that a patient's cancer has spread beyond the original tumor site, the message to the physician and patient is clear: the cancer has metastasized, and systemic therapy is likely going to be required.

However, a more difficult situation arises when staging studies do not detect cancer cells beyond the original tumor site. The physician must remember that, while staging studies are powerful, and becoming more powerful as the technologies advance, they do have detection limits—they cannot find everything, everywhere in the body. Additionally, with regard to sentinel lymph node testing, not all cancer spreads through the lymph nodes, so, while this is a good way to determine whether a cancer is metastatic, it will not detect all metastatic disease.[1]

What do the physician and patient do when staging studies are negative? In these cases, the physician has to estimate the likelihood that cancer cells have, in fact, spread to other parts of the body but are, at the time, so few in number that they cannot be detected by the testing methods used.

Asking how likely it is that a cancer has spread is a vitally important question because, if the cancer has metastasized despite the negative findings, the metastases will not stay small. And, if metastases are not dealt with early, while they are still small, they may be much harder to treat later, once they have grown and spread further.

As a medical oncologist, it has been my experience that most cancers are already systemic at the time they are diagnosed. This is because cancer can go undetected for months or years before a patient begins to show symptoms, allowing plenty of time for a tumor to metastasize before it is diagnosed. If I only pay attention to the original tumor, and put too much confidence in negative staging studies, without considering the possibility of metastatic disease, I risk having my patients return to my clinic months or years after their initial treatment with a far more advanced cancer than was originally diagnosed.

But systemic therapies are not without their own risks and side effects, and I do not want to subject my patients to risks and adverse side effects unnecessarily. So, I must carefully consider the cancer involved in each case. Doctors know that some types of cancer are far more likely to metastasize than others, and some are far more likely to metastasize before they begin to show symptoms. When developing a treatment plan for my patients, I always take into consideration the type of cancer each patient has and the possibility that the cancer has already metastasized at the time of diagnosis. In this way, I can better assess the risks and benefits of moving ahead with systemic therapy for my patients.

∾

When a decision is made to go forward with systemic therapy, the physician has many forms of systemic therapy from which to choose, including chemotherapy, immunotherapy, biological therapy, hormone therapy and targeted therapy. Many cancer patients require systemic therapy in combination with surgery and radiation therapy, and some patients may need more than one type of systemic therapy. For some accessible and reliable online reading material on the different types of systemic therapy, see the notes for this chapter.[2-12]

~

The most commonly used form of systemic therapy is chemo-therapy.[2] Chemotherapy, commonly called chemo, uses drugs to attack cancer cells. Chemotherapy drugs are designed to accelerate cell death in rapidly dividing cells, and these drugs take advantage of the fact that cancer cells are usually rapidly dividing. Chemotherapy can be used to shrink a primary tumor, kill cancer cells that have spread from the original tumor site, kill cancer cells not removed by surgery or destroyed by radiation therapy, reduce symptoms caused by cancer or treat a recurrence of cancer.

Depending upon the type and stage of your cancer, your doctor may have many chemotherapy drugs from which to choose. Sometimes physicians use a combination of chemotherapy drugs to treat patients. The reason for this is that the mechanism of action—the cellular pathways on which a drug works—can differ from drug to drug. By using a mixture of drugs, doctors can attack different cellular pathways in cancer cells at the same time. It is like a one-two punch, and, in some cases, it is more effective at killing cancer cells than any one drug can be on its own.

Chemotherapy can be administered in a number of different ways. Some chemotherapy drugs are oral medications (taken by mouth), some are topical (rubbed onto the skin) and some are injected in the form of a shot. Some chemotherapy drugs are delivered intravenously or intra-arterially, by inserting a tube directly into a vein or artery, or intraperitoneally—introduced directly into the abdominal cavity.

Unfortunately, there is still one place in the body that chemo-therapy drugs cannot reach effectively: the brain. This is because of the blood-brain barrier which stops many medications from getting to the brain. Typically, only small amounts of chemotherapy drugs get across the blood-brain barrier and into the brain—usually not enough to be effective against the cancer. Of course, some drugs are better than others at crossing the blood-brain barrier, but many are essentially stopped. Sometimes, chemotherapy drugs that need to get to the brain are administered by a method called intrathecal injection—an injection directly into the spinal canal.

Chemotherapy is a long-term treatment, usually given over a period of weeks. Some patients might be given chemotherapy in cycles that consist of a week of daily chemotherapy followed by a rest period of two to three weeks before the cycle is started again. The rest period allows the body to recover from the chemotherapy treatment and prepare for the next cycle.

It is important to remember that each cancer, and each cancer patient, will respond to chemotherapy differently. Your treating physician or medical oncologist will evaluate you regularly to see how you are responding to the drugs. This evaluation may include imaging studies to see if chemotherapy has shrunk your tumor, or blood work to assess tumor and other markers. Based on the findings of these studies and any side effects that you may have, your doctor might adjust the dose of chemotherapy drugs you will receive in the next cycle of treatment.

～

Immunotherapy is another form of systemic therapy that is some-times used in the fight against cancer. Immunotherapy takes many forms. One form of immunotherapy involves giving antibodies to cancer patients. Antibodies are proteins made by the immune system to help the body fight against infection. Antibodies can also be grown in the laboratory in large quantities, and can bind to their targets with very high specificity.[3-6]

Antibody therapy for cancer sometimes uses antibodies that recognize and bind specific targets on cancer cells. In one form of antibody therapy, antibodies are used to tag cancer cells for destruction by the immune system. For example, the antibody alemtuzumab, also known as Campath, binds to a specific protein on lymphocytes (a type of white blood cell), marking these cells for destruction by the immune system. Alemtuzumab is used in the treatment of chronic lymphocytic leukemia (CLL).

Antibodies can also be used to bind specific targets on cancer cells in order to block the cellular signals that encourage cancer cells to divide. For example, the antibody trastuzumab, also known as Herceptin, binds to a protein on breast and stomach cancer cells called HER2. Trastuzumab blocks the ability of the HER2 protein to tell cancer cells to divide.

Antibodies can also be designed to interrupt the normal inhibitory signals that, in the absence of cancer, help keep the immune system under control. As Dr. Teh discussed briefly in the previous chapter, this type of immunotherapy stimulates the immune system, so that it can attack cancer cells. For example, nivolumab, also known as Opdivo; pembrolizumab, also known as Keytruda; and ipilimumab, also known as Yervoy, are all antibodies that block inhibitory signals in the immune system. These antibodies are used in the treatment of melanoma. Nivolumab and pembrolizumab are also used in the treatment of non-small cell lung cancer and other types of cancer.

Antibodies can also be designed to deliver toxins, radioactive compounds or drugs to cancer cells. In this method, antibodies that target cancer cells are tagged with compounds which kill cells.

Another type of immunotherapy involves giving patients substances that elevate the overall level of activity of the immune system. In one form of this type of immunotherapy, cytokines—substances that activate immune cells, such as interferons or interleukins, or other immune stimulating drugs—are given to patients. These drugs boost the immune system and stimulate the immune cells that recognize cancer cells.[3,7,8]

Another form of immunotherapy involves giving patients a weakened bacterium called Bacillus Calmette-Guérin or BCG. The bacteria are placed at the site of the tumor to stimulate an immune response against both the bacteria and the cancer. BCG is currently used to treat bladder cancer and melanoma, but its use in treating other types of cancer is being investigated.[3,7,8]

Other types of immunotherapy for cancer include vaccines that prevent or treat cancer and cellular therapies in which a sample of a patient's immune cells are taken from the body, modulated in the laboratory and given back to the patient to heighten the immune system's ability to attack and destroy the cancer.[3,4,9]

Like chemotherapy, immunotherapy may be given in cycles that include a period of treatment followed by a period without treatment. Immunotherapy may also be given according to other schedules, depending upon the type and stage of cancer and the immunotherapy being used. As with chemotherapy, your doctor will monitor you regularly for side effects to see how you are reacting to the treatment and to consider whether your treatment needs to be adjusted.

∿

Biological therapy for cancer uses substances derived from biological organisms. These substances act in a variety of ways to treat cancer.[3,7] For example, immunotherapies that use antibodies, cytokines, immune cells and bacteria are examples of biological therapies for cancer.

Another biological therapy for cancer is gene therapy. In one common method of performing gene therapy, viruses are modified in the laboratory to remove many of the viral genes and incorporate sequences of DNA or RNA that have been specifically engineered for therapeutic purposes. The modified viruses are given to patients so that they can infect cancer cells, inserting the engineered sequences of DNA or RNA into the infected cells. Because the modified viruses lack the genes needed for the virus to replicate itself, the modified viruses cannot continue to infect new cells; they are only good for a single round of infection that delivers the engineered DNA or RNA. After infection, the engineered DNA or RNA is used by infected cells to manufacture proteins that would not otherwise exist in the cancer cells, but that can now be exploited to slow the growth of cancer cells, stimulate the immune system against the cancer cells or make the cancer cells more susceptible to cytotoxic treatments, such as medications or radiation therapy.

～

Hormone therapy is another type of systemic therapy for cancer. Hormone therapy works because some cancers, like prostate and breast cancer, need hormones in order to grow. Hormone therapy deprives the cancer cells of the hormones they need, limiting the ability of the cancer cells to multiply. Hormone therapy can include surgery to remove hormone-producing organs, such as the testicles or ovaries, or medications to block the production or action of hormones within the body.[13,14]

For example, early-stage prostate cancer cells are stimulated by androgens (male sex hormones) such as testosterone. The goal of hormone therapy for prostate cancer is to eliminate the effects of androgens on cancer cells. To achieve this goal, doctors have several options. Surgeons can perform surgery to remove the testicles, a procedure called orchiectomy or orchidectomy. This surgery will greatly reduce the amount of testosterone in the body. Doctors can also prescribe medications to block the production of testosterone by the testicles. Drugs such as goserelin (also called Zoladex), leuprolide (also called Lupron), and degarelix prevent the production of testosterone by blocking the signaling pathway that tells the body to make testosterone. Some drugs such as ketoconazole and others interfere with the production of testosterone by other cells in the body, including the cells of the adrenal glands and prostate cancer cells. Ketoconazole, and drugs similar to it, work by inhibiting one of the enzymes required for the production of testosterone, blocking the biochemical pathway that manufactures testosterone.

Another option doctors have for hormone therapy against prostate cancer is to prescribe drugs that interrupt the ability of androgens to tell prostate cancer cells to multiply. Drugs such as flutamide, nilutamide and others bind the androgen receptor proteins found in prostate cancer cells and occupy the receptor so that androgens cannot bind. The interference by the drug inhibits the ability of androgens to tell the prostate cancer cells to multiply.

Often, several drugs will be used together in the treatment of prostate cancer. Hormone therapy for prostate cancer may be given before or after other cancer treatments such as surgery or radiation therapy, and may also be given to patients who have had a recurrence or metastasis of their prostate cancer.

Just as prostate cancer cells can be stimulated by testosterone, some types of breast cancer cells are stimulated by the female sex hormone: estrogen. In order to eliminate the effects of estrogen on breast cancer cells, doctors can use an approach called ovarian ablation where either surgery is performed to remove the ovaries, a procedure called oophorectomy, or radiation treatments are given to suppress ovarian function. Doctors can also use medications that inhibit the production of estrogen by the ovaries. Two such drugs, goserelin and leuprolide, block the signaling pathway that tells the body to make estrogen. Other drugs such as anastrozole, also called Arimidex, and exemestane, also called Aromasin, interfere with the manufacture of estrogen in the ovaries and in other tissues that also make estrogen, including fat and skin cells. These drugs work by inhibiting an enzyme required for the production of estrogen.

Another option doctors have is to prescribe drugs that interrupt the ability of estrogen to tell breast cancer cells to multiply. Drugs such as tamoxifen, also called Nolvadex; raloxifene, also called Evista; and fulvestrant, also called Faslodex, bind to estrogen receptors on breast cancer cells and occupy the receptor so that estrogen cannot bind.

Often several drugs will be used together in the treatment of breast cancer. Hormone therapy for breast cancer is often given in combination with other cancer treatments, such as surgery or radiation therapy, or to patients who have metastatic breast cancer.

∼

Targeted therapy for cancer is based on a specific characteristic unique to a particular cancer, such as a discrete genetic change, a distinct immunologic feature or a need for hormones. For example, in contrast to the most commonly used chemotherapy drugs, such as doxorubicin HCL, also called Adriamycin, or cyclophosphamide that act on both cancerous and non-cancerous cells, targeted therapy works by going after a characteristic that is unique to the particular type of cancer cell it is designed to attack. Because non-cancerous cells do not have the characteristic the therapy is designed to attack, targeted therapy endeavors to minimize the effect on non-cancerous cells. The goal of targeted therapy is to compromise the cancer cells by impeding their ability to multiply, enhancing the destruction or death of cancer cells, or inhibiting angiogenesis—the growth of new blood vessels which feed the tumors. [11,15,16]

One frequently used targeted therapy is imatinib mesylate, also called Gleevec. Imatinib mesylate binds to specific proteins found in chronic myeloid leukemia (CML) cells, acute lymphocytic leukemia (ALL) cells and the cells of a few other cancers. In the case of CML and ALL cells, it is the protein called BCR-ABL that is recognized by imatinib mesylate. The BCR-ABL protein does not exist in non-CML or non-ALL cells, so imatinib mesylate leaves non-CML and non-ALL cells alone. When imatinib mesylate binds to the BCR-ABL protein, it prevents BCR-ABL from telling the CML or ALL cells to multiply. [15,16]

～

There is considerable overlap between the different forms of systemic therapy. Some therapies may simultaneously be immunological, biological and targeted or simultaneously chemotherapy and targeted. For example, immunotherapies are typically biological therapies that are often also targeted therapies. Hormone therapies are often targeted therapies. Additionally, some chemotherapy drugs are designed specifically to attack particular genetic changes that occur in cancer, making them also targeted therapies. This is sometimes called precision medicine. If your doctor is considering giving you a targeted chemotherapy drug, genetic testing of your cancer may be required in order to determine whether these drugs are right for you.[11,12]

~

Systemic therapies for cancer can be quite effective but these therapies are not without side effects. In fact, side effects are a frequent problem in systemic therapy. The types of side effects that can occur depend upon the type of therapy being used and the dose.[2,3,10,17]

The reason systemic therapy is associated with side effects is that the treatment is delivered to the whole body. And while it may be particularly good at harming cancer cells, it may also harm healthy cells and compromise the function of non-cancerous tissues and organs. The side effects of systemic therapy vary from person to person, according to the therapy given, and can range from mild to severe.

Some of the side effects commonly seen in patients receiving chemotherapy include an increased risk of infection, fatigue, nausea, vomiting, hair loss, diarrhea, constipation, easy bruising or bleeding and sores in the mouth.[2,17]

Side effects can also occur with immunotherapy for cancer.[3,6,8] Side effects from immunotherapy can include swelling, irritation, a rash or soreness at injection sites and flu-like symptoms. Immunotherapy may also cause an increased risk of infection, cough, congestion, diarrhea and rapid, strong or irregular heartbeat. Immunotherapy for cancer can also cause allergic reactions that may be life-threatening.

Depending upon the type of hormone therapy received, side effects of hormone therapy can include hot flashes, loss of libido, sexual dysfunction, mood changes, fatigue, nausea, diarrhea, changes in menstruation and changes in bone density.[10]

Even targeted therapies can cause side effects.[11] The side effects seen with targeted therapy typically depend upon the type of therapy and the target but can include fatigue, sores in the mouth, skin problems, diarrhea and several other problems.

～

Now that you have learned in the last few chapters about the three major approaches to treating cancer: surgery, radiation therapy and systemic therapy, let's discuss how doctors manage the various side effects of these treatments with medical supportive therapy.

9

MEDICAL SUPPORTIVE THERAPY

Although medicines can make you feel better and help you get well, it's
important to know that ALL medicines... have risks as well as benefits.

FOOD AND DRUG ADMINISTRATION,
U.S. DEPARTMENT OF HEALTH AND HUMAN SERVICES[1]

The general practice of monitoring and working to reduce the impacts of cancer and cancer treatment on patients is called medical supportive therapy or supportive care. You may recall we discussed medical supportive therapy briefly in Chapters 4 and 6. In this chapter, I will go deeper into this topic.

~

Medical supportive therapy has two objectives: to control the complications of cancer and cancer treatment and to make the quality of life of a cancer patient as normal as possible. The first objective seeks to minimize the negative impacts of cancer and its treatment. At first glance, you may think this is mostly about controlling the side effects of cancer treatment, but it is important to remember that cancer itself can cause side effects, including many of the same side effects that are caused by treatment.

The second objective of medical supportive therapy deals with quality-of-life issues, and is concerned with improving the general health, comfort, happiness, sense of well-being and degree of satisfaction patients feel in the course of daily life. Both cancer and its treatment can have a huge impact on a patient's quality of life. Patients may feel sick, uncomfortable, self-conscious, anxious, frightened and less secure in their sense of well-being. They may be fearful for the future and have less joy and satisfaction in the activities of living.

I believe that medical supportive therapy is a critically important part of caring for my patients. When patients feel better, they have a more positive outlook and are better prepared to deal with challenges, whether related to cancer, its treatment or day-to-day living. Patients who feel better are also more likely to participate in their own treatment and take care of themselves, preserving dignity and self-reliance. I also find that patients who feel better are far less likely to stop treatment, and far more likely to participate in the activities they enjoy, such as going to work, going shopping and spending time with friends and loved ones.

～

The side effects of cancer and cancer treatment vary from person to person based on the type of cancer a person has, the types and combinations of treatments received and the physical differences that naturally exist between people. Fortunately, patients do not have to endure many of the side effects of cancer and its treatment, because physicians have powerful weapons to fight these side effects.[2]

A full discussion of the potential side effects of every type of cancer and every type of treatment used to fight cancer would fill several books. Here, I will mention only a few of the most common side effects of cancer and cancer treatment and highlight some of the ways and means doctors have to manage them. For a more personalized discussion of the potential side effects of your cancer and the treatments you will receive in the course of your cancer care, I urge you to talk to your doctor.

∾

An increased risk of infection is the most serious side effect of cancer and cancer treatment.[3-6] In fact, infections in cancer patients are usually considered a medical emergency because they can quickly become life-threatening.

The increased risk of infection occurs in cancer patients because of a reduction in the number of white blood cells, particularly a special type of white blood cell called neutrophils. Neutrophils are a critical part of the body's defenses against infection. When a person has a low level of neutrophils in their blood it is called neutropenia. Cancer patients develop neutropenia because some cancers, and some cancer treatments such as chemotherapy or radiation therapy, affect the bone marrow— the substance inside bones that makes blood cells. Sometimes, a person with neutropenia is referred to as being immunocompromised.

The pathogens that cause infections, and the symptoms of infection, in cancer patients are often similar to the pathogens and symptoms in people without cancer, but cancer patients may be particularly susceptible to infection by pathogens that do not normally cause disease in people without cancer. To reduce your risk of infection during cancer treatment, practice good hygiene, avoid injuries, pay attention to food safety and avoid germs found in crowds and people who have recently been sick, i.e. with the common cold or flu.

Fortunately, doctors have a variety of medications that can help prevent infection in cancer patients. Some of these medications boost the immune system by helping the body make more white blood cells, including neutrophils. Physicians often prescribe these medications very early in the treatment of cancer patients because they want to stop, and reverse, the decline in the levels of neutrophils in a patient's blood, before an infection occurs. The medications used to fight neutropenia are called growth factors or colony-stimulating factors (CSFs) and include drugs such as peg-filgrastim, also called Neulasta; filgrastim, also called Neupogen; and sargramostim, also called Leukine.

Sometimes, cancer patients are also given prophylactic (preventive) antibiotics to help reduce the risk of infection. Although this approach cannot prevent all infections in cancer patients, it can make cancer patients less likely to get an infection while their neutrophils are low.

～

Fatigue is one of the most common problems faced by cancer patients.[7-12] Fatigue can be caused, or worsened, by many things including the cancer itself, cancer treatments, depression and the powerful emotions and stress that occur as a result of a serious illness such as cancer. Lack of sleep, nutritional deficits and other medical problems in addition to cancer can also cause fatigue.

Each of these causes of fatigue require different approaches to treatment, but there are plenty of treatment options. If you have fatigue, I urge you to talk to your doctor to investigate the cause of your fatigue and develop an effective management plan. It is also important, no matter the cause of your fatigue, that you get plenty of rest but also remain active and get proper nutrition.

The most common cause of fatigue in cancer patients is anemia—reduction in the number of red blood cells. Red blood cells carry oxygen to the tissues of the body. When tissues do not get enough oxygen, feelings of fatigue and weakness can result. Anemia can also cause pallor (extreme paleness), shortness of breath, rapid heartbeat, dizziness, headaches, chest pain and swelling in the hands or feet. In cancer patients, anemia often occurs when cancer and cancer treatment affect the bone marrow.

Fortunately, doctors have a number of choices when it comes to treating anemia in cancer patients. Blood transfusions are one option that can provide a fresh supply of red blood cells very quickly. There are also medications available for treating anemia. Drugs such as epoetin, also called Procrit or Epogen; and darbepoetin, also called Aranesp, boost the production of red blood cells and can help with the symptoms of fatigue.

Pain is another factor that can also substantially affect the quality of life of cancer patients.[13,14] The pain felt by cancer patients may be caused by the cancer itself or by cancer treatments. For example, tumors can cause pain if they stimulate surrounding nerve cells. Also, diagnostic procedures and surgery for cancer can cause pain, and radiation therapy for cancer can have painful side effects, including burns, scars, sores or injury to delicate tissues. Systemic therapies such as chemotherapy can also have painful side effects. One example is the mouth sores caused by certain chemotherapy drugs.

Fortunately, doctors can use a number of different medications to manage pain. There are also drug-free therapies for managing pain such as acupuncture, biofeedback and others. No matter what treatment is prescribed to manage your pain, it is important that you follow the treatment plan laid out by your doctor.

If you are prescribed medications for your pain, take your medications as directed by your physician. If you cannot take your pain medication on time, or if you take less medicine than prescribed, your pain may persist. But pain medication is potent medicine, so taking your medication too often, or taking too much, can cause serious or even life-threatening reactions. If you are feeling pain that bothers you, interferes with your daily life, affects your ability to eat or sleep or compromises your ability or willingness to do the things you want to do, I urge you to talk to your doctor about managing your pain. Your doctor may decide to include a pain specialist in your care team. Pain specialists are doctors specifically trained to manage pain.

$\sim$

Nausea and vomiting are also common problems for cancer patients and, like pain, these can have a huge impact on a patient's quality of life.[15,16] They can be caused by the cancer itself or by cancer treatments, including chemotherapy and radiation therapy. They can also be caused by bowel disturbances, infections, electrolyte imbalances and other problems.

Nausea and vomiting affect a patient's willingness to eat and drink as well as their ability to keep down food and liquids that are ingested. They can lead to weight loss, and, in severe cases, dehydration, electrolyte imbalances and malnutrition. Nausea and vomiting can also lead to feelings of fatigue and interfere with wound healing or the ability to take medications by mouth.

Fortunately, there are a variety of anti-nausea medications that can help.[17] These medications are called anti-emetics. A wide variety of anti-emetics exist, and they act in different ways to prevent nausea and vomiting. But not all drugs work for all people. It can take a bit of trial and error to find the best medicine for you, and you may need to take more than one medicine at a time, but be persistent. It is important to keep nausea and vomiting under control so that you eat and drink as normally as possible and maintain your nutrition, strength and weight.

There are also many things cancer patients can do for themselves to improve nausea and vomiting including avoiding greasy, spicy or sweet foods, eating smaller quantities more often and making an effort to get enough fluids. Again, drug-free therapies such as acupuncture, biofeedback and others can help.[15,18]

Cancer and cancer treatments can also affect the number of platelets in the blood.[19] Platelets are cells that help stop bleeding. When a person has low platelets, it is called thrombocytopenia. People with this condition may bruise easily and are at risk of excessive bleeding.

Cancer patients with thrombocytopenia need to be careful about things that can cause bleeding, including excessively dry skin, chapping or injury. Be careful to avoid bumping into things or falling, and avoid certain medications that can increase risk of bleeding. Even activities as common as brushing your teeth, cutting yourself with a razor, scissors or a knife and constipation can lead to serious bleeding in a cancer patient with thrombocytopenia.

Depending on the kind of cancer you have, and the treatments you are receiving, your care team can advise you about your risk of bleeding and any precautions you should take to avoid a bleeding event.

∾

When I discuss medical supportive therapy with my patients, I always keep in mind that all medications used in medical supportive therapy can have side effects of their own, and some pain medications can be addictive. Before you begin medical supportive therapy, I urge you to talk to your doctor about your treatment options, your medical history, all of the medications you take and your experiences with medications you have taken in the past. I also urge you to talk to your doctor about possible side effects or risks associated with any medications you might be considering and how those side effects and risks will be managed.

∾

Proper nutrition is also an important part of medical supportive therapy during cancer treatment.[20,21] A good diet will help with fatigue and with your body's response to treatment, ability to fight cancer and capacity to heal. Proper nutrition will also help you feel better, keep up your weight and stamina and enhance your ability to fight infection and deal with the side effects of treatments.

A good diet involves getting enough of the right kinds of calories and nutrients to keep your body functioning optimally. This includes proteins, fats, carbohydrates and water. But eating properly during cancer treatment can be a challenge. You may feel nauseated or just not hungry. Food may not smell or taste the same. And your ability to digest foods or absorb nutrients from food may be altered.

Cancer patients may also have particular nutritional needs that might need attention, beyond simply a good healthy diet. You may need to consume more calories or more of certain types of foods than you normally would, or eat foods that are easy to ingest and digest or are soothing to the mouth and gastrointestinal tract. There may be foods you need to make sure you eat and foods you need to avoid based on the treatments and medications you receive. You may need to handle and prepare your food in certain ways. There also may be herbs and supplements you should take and herbs and supplements you should avoid, depending upon your treatments.

Your doctor can help you understand your nutritional requirements during treatment and how they may differ from time to time based upon the type of cancer you have and the types of treatments you are receiving. Your doctor may also connect you with a nutritionist to help you plan and monitor your diet and weight.

But assuring good nutrition is not just the responsibility of your doctor or nutritionist. Good nutrition requires your involvement. I recommend that my patients eat good quality food and avoid junk food or fast food. I recommend they reduce their salt, sugar and alcohol intake, avoid spicy foods that can irritate the digestive tract and eliminate raw foods that may increase the chance of food-borne infections. I also suggest my patients avoid canned foods and foods with preservatives. Finally, I recommend they make a point of eating regularly, but not too much at one time.

For patients having particular difficulty eating, doctors may need to provide supplemental nutritional support, such as enteral or parenteral nutrition. Enteral nutrition, also called tube feeding, provides nutrition in liquid form. Tubes may be passed through the nose and throat or placed directly into the stomach or small intestine through a hole in the abdomen. Once placed, nutrition is delivered through the tube. Parenteral nutrition also delivers nutrients in liquid form, but bypasses the stomach and intestines and delivers nutrition through a catheter (a thin tube) inserted into a vein. In this way, nutrients are introduced directly into the blood.

∼

Unfortunately, not all treatment facilities have the resources to provide medical supportive therapy. If you are being treated in a facility that does not offer medical supportive therapy, I recommend that you talk to your doctor about the types of supportive therapy you might need and where you might be able to get that therapy.

You may have to advocate for yourself, but, in my experience, medical supportive therapy is very important. Without it, your quality of life may be compromised and your desire to fight your cancer can be impacted. I urge you to do what you can to get the supportive therapy you need to stay as strong and comfortable as possible during your cancer treatments.

∼

Another kind of supportive therapy for cancer may not necessarily involve the prescription of medications by a physician, but is no less important for quality of life. This type of supportive care focuses on a patient's psychological outlook and deals with matters related to emotional issues, worries, fears and the challenges of day-to-day living.

Not all cancer patients need this type of supportive care, but patients who receive additional psychological supportive care may experience an improved outlook, more hope for the future and a greater willingness to keep up the long, often psychologically and emotionally taxing, fight against cancer.

For some cancer patients keeping up the fight is all it takes. New treatments for cancer are always becoming available. It is important to remember that just because there may not be a treatment for your type of cancer today, it does not mean there won't be a treatment tomorrow, or next month, or next year. So, keeping up the fight could mean surviving until a better, more effective treatment comes along.

Now that you have learned about the different types of medical supportive therapy that are available, let's talk about the power of hope, perseverance, love and compassion.

10

THE POWER OF HOPE, PERSEVERANCE, LOVE AND COMPASSION

Hope is the thing with feathers
That perches in the soul,
And sings the tune without the words,
And never stops at all...

EMILY DICKINSON[1]

Give us grace and strength to forbear and to persevere.

ROBERT LOUIS STEVENSON[2]

Love conquers all; let us, too, yield to Love!

VIRGIL[3]

As we have discussed in the last few chapters, treatment is important for cancer patients. But cancer patients need much more than procedures and medications; they also need hope, perseverance, love and compassion.

∼

The Merriam-Webster Dictionary defines hope as "to cherish a desire with anticipation" and perseverance as a "continued effort to do or achieve something despite difficulties, failure, or opposition".

While hope is important in many aspects of life, it is essential for the cancer patient, because hope fuels perseverance. Without hope, cancer patients can fall into despair and lose perseverance. Without perseverance, cancer patients can lose the will to fight.

Cancer treatment can be a long road, and it is not always a straight line. There may be progress, but there may also be setbacks. Hope and perseverance will keep you going forward, keep you fighting. Even if there is not a cure for your cancer today, there may be treatments that can provide a normal quality of life and prolong your life until a new treatment may offer the chance for a cure. If you give up on your treatment after the first, second or any subsequent setback, you may never get to that chance for a cure.

Hope comes from many sources. Family and friends are important, but patients also look to their doctors for hope. In American medicine today, however, there is a tendency not to pay much attention to hope. Doctors often become so consumed with the physical aspects of a patient's disease and the logistics of treatment that they do not give much thought or time to addressing the psychological state of the patient.

Further, some doctors may not be skilled in communicating with patients in a way that preserves hope. As a result, doctors can strip their patients of hope. Not intentionally perhaps, but when a doctor rushes through patient visits and focuses solely on the negative or problematic aspects of a patient's cancer, transmitting information in a way that lacks tact or is pessimistic about the future, patients can lose hope.

I work hard to provide patient care in a manner that preserves hope. It just takes conscious recognition of what the patient is going through, sensitivity in communicating and time. The unfortunate reality is that doctors do not often have time to give

Nigel's story

Nigel has non-Hodgkin's lymphoma. He was treated for two years in his home country but did not respond. His doctors considered him to be terminal.

So, Nigel came to the United States to seek treatment. He saw various doctors at various institutions around the country. None believed Nigel had a chance for a cure. But Nigel did not give up. He continued to be hopeful and kept his perseverance. This led Nigel to me.

I started Nigel on a treatment regimen that included drugs he had not previously received. After one month of treatment, 60-70 percent of Nigel's disease had been eradicated. With this kind of response to treatment, Nigel now has a chance to be cured. This is because patients with non-Hodgkin's lymphoma who respond like this to treatment have a reasonable chance for cure.

As a result of our success against his cancer, Nigel is a different person to the man who came to see me just a few short weeks earlier. He is now asymptomatic and leading a normal life. He is eating well, his energy has returned, and he is enjoying life once again. Were it not for his hope and perseverance, Nigel would have died.

patients the lengthy conversations that provide comfort and compassion, alleviate anxiety, infuse courage, and support a positive, hopeful attitude.

In my practice, I am lucky to be able to provide my patients with my time and access to me. However, many patients will not have a physician who can offer time and access. If you find yourself in this position, I urge you to advocate for yourself and talk to your doctor about what you need. If your doctor is unable to provide the resources you require, ask where you might find resources that can help you maintain your hope and perseverance.

~

The Merriam-Webster Dictionary offers several definitions of love but the most relevant to our discussion here is "unselfish loyal and benevolent concern for the good of another".

Love is a powerful weapon in the fight against cancer. Along with hope, love gives us courage and makes us feel valuable and needed. Patients who feel they do not have love may feel all alone in the battle against cancer and may find it difficult to maintain hope.

In my experience, an important source of love in cancer care is the love of doctors and nurses. Doctors and nurses who truly feel love for their patients are more inclined to demonstrate empathy, be concerned with how their patients are doing every day and listen intently, really hearing what patients are saying. Doctors and nurses who love their patients are better equipped to go the extra mile for them and to provide the patience and care that convey love. They are also less likely to give up on their patients.

In the United States, however, there is a general sense that doctors and nurses should keep an emotional distance or be detached from their patients. For some diseases this may not matter, but, in cancer care, patients need to feel close to their doctors and nurses. This is because cancer patients often feel that their lives are threatened by their disease. They need to feel that their doctors and nurses love and care for them and are really trying to save them. For this reason, I believe that in cancer care the emotional

Owen's story

Many years ago, before coming to the United States, I had a patient we'll call Owen. Owen had hairy cell leukemia. At the time, there was no treatment for this disease.

I suggested to Owen that he travel to America to consult with doctors at a major cancer center. He did this, but the doctors told him to go home and live out what was left of his life because there was no treatment for his cancer, and they could not save him.

When Owen got home, he came to see me and asked me to help him commit suicide. He did not want to go through the long, painful illness that he anticipated. He had given up.

But I sat with Owen. I told him how much I loved him as a person and explained how I could treat him with standard therapy, not with the goal of curing his cancer, but with the goal of prolonging his life in the hope that a new drug might be available one day to cure his cancer.

It took several hours to convince Owen to accept my plea. Finally, he said he would do this for me, because he now understood how traumatic it would be for me if he committed suicide.

We started Owen on the standard treatment that was available at the time. Two years later, a new drug became available that was capable of curing most patients with hairy cell leukemia. By then, I was in the United States, so Owen came to America for this new treatment. More than thirty years later, Owen is still alive and his cancer has never returned.

distance between doctors and nurses and their patients should be as short as possible.

Fortunately, love does not require much time. Love can be found in every interaction and communication. However, the pressures that plague the practice of medicine today can create an environment that drains the capacity to love from health care workers.

This is where family and friends can help. Ideally, family and friends are nearby and can be with, and support, you every day. However, in today's complex society, friends and family may not always be nearby, especially if you must travel to receive cancer treatment. Although not a substitute for being there, computers and smartphones can help you stay connected to family and friends.

∽

The Merriam-Webster Dictionary defines compassion as "sympathetic consciousness of others' distress together with a desire to alleviate it".

Compassion is also important to the cancer patient. It touches cancer patients in a way that is difficult to define, but it lessens suffering, pain and feelings of isolation. Offering effective compassion requires seeing the human being behind the disease and appreciating the patient as a person. Without this capacity, compassion is compromised.

Doctors get a great deal of training in medical procedures and treatment, but they do not often get much training in the art of expressing compassion for their patients. As a result, some doctors may feel that providing compassion is not their job—their only job is to treat disease.

The consequence of this approach is that the focus of the doctor is on the cold, clinical aspects of disease, without attending

Paula's story

One day, several years ago, I was making rounds in the hospital and saw Paula. Paula was in her thirties and had breast cancer. When I stopped by Paula's room, she was crying. She had been told that her disease was incurable and there was no sense in receiving further treatment since there was no chance for a cure. Based on this opinion from her doctors, Paula decided to stop treatment for her cancer.

I sat with Paula for a long time, listened to her fears and concerns, heard her hopelessness and desperation, and just held her hands. She came to realize that I understood what she was feeling and sympathized with the agony she was in. She had two small children and feared what might happen to them once she was gone. But the more we talked, and the more I explained to her that, while it was true that her disease was incurable at this time, I might be able to prolong her life, giving her the chance to receive a new treatment that might become available one day if she could just find the hope and perseverance to continue treatment.

After spending time with Paula, and giving her the compassion she needed to find hope again, she agreed to continue treatment. Today, more than ten years later, Paula is still alive. She is not free of the disease, but she is alive, asymptomatic, and leading a normal life, with a normal quality of life. She still gets treatment for her cancer, but she has been able to watch her children grow and be a part of their lives.

to the human being affected by the disease. This leads patients to feel that their medical team does not care about them or their success against cancer.

If you feel your treatment team lacks sufficient loyal and benevolent concern for you, family and friends can provide compassion. As we discussed in the previous section, ideally you will have your family and friends nearby while you are being treated for cancer. If not, I urge you to use the communications technologies available to you to stay in touch.

～

One of the biggest obstacles to hope, perseverance, love and compassion in medicine today is the corporatization of medical practice and the focus on the financial aspects of patient care. In my experience, it is extraordinarily difficult to commercialize medicine without losing the human side of the endeavor. But when we sacrifice the human side of medicine, we strip patient care of the love and compassion needed to maintain hope and perseverance. And, while this may not be so important to the patient with a simple fracture or earache, it is critical for the cancer patient.

If you feel that love and compassion are absent from your cancer care, and you do not have friends and family nearby to provide the support you need, I urge you to talk to your doctor about patient support groups, psychological support or other resources that can help you maintain hope and perseverance. Support groups can be helpful because they bring patients together to share common experiences, concerns and fears. These groups often provide a sense of community and lessen feelings of fighting cancer all alone. Individuals in support groups frequently become a close-knit group, loving and caring for one another, celebrating victories together and supporting each other through difficult times. These benefits of support groups fuel hope, courage and perseverance for the individuals in the group.

But support groups are not for everyone. Fortunately, support groups are not the only alternative for finding love and compassion in the course of your cancer treatment. If you feel you need additional support, but choose not to participate in a support group, advocate for yourself. Talk to your doctor about other resources that may be available to provide you with the support, love and compassion that you need. You may need to search for a while to find the support you need, but it will be time well spent.

∼

Now that we've discussed the power of hope, perseverance, love and compassion, let's talk about quality of life.

11

QUALITY OF LIFE

*We've been wrong about what our job is in medicine. We think
our job is to ensure health and survival. But really it is larger
than that. It is to enable well-being. And well-being is about the
reasons one wishes to be alive. Those reasons matter not just at
the end of life, or when debility comes, but all along the way.*

ATUL GAWANDE, M.D., M.P.H. [1]

In American society today, there is a great deal of discussion about
quality of life in the context of end-of-life care and how people
wish to spend their last days, weeks or months. I see it all the
time—people only really thinking or talking about quality-of-life
issues in times of illness or when they are close to death.

But, in my years of medical practice, I have come to believe
that each of us should think about our personal quality of life long
before the end of our days. It is far more important to have a good
quality of life throughout one's life. I believe people should make
conscious decisions to ensure quality of life. This means orienting
themselves early on in life toward caring for their personal health
and well-being.

One way to care for one's quality of life involves reducing the
risk of disease. Do not take your health for granted. Get regular
checkups and address signs and symptoms of disease early. Do not

engage thoughtlessly in risky behaviors that can cause injury or illness. Do not smoke, take illegal drugs or misuse legal drugs and prescription medications. Exercise, eat a healthy diet, get enough sleep and take steps to reduce stress.

Another way to care for your quality of life involves attending to your emotional and psychological well-being. Develop and maintain a supportive network of family and friends. Engage thoughtfully and caringly with those around you. Participate in activities that give you joy and bring meaning to your life. Live fully in each moment and embrace life in all its wonder. Actively seek to maintain a positive outlook and derive satisfaction from life.

~

Having said that, my professional experience lies mostly with patients and families discussing quality-of-life issues in the context of serious illness. The problem I see all too often is that my patients and their loved ones are lured by the misconception that, in the context of cancer, it is better to have quality of life than it is to pursue a treatment such as chemotherapy, surgery or radiation therapy which might make the patient miserable.

But there are two major flaws in this reasoning: the mistaken belief that quality of life can be achieved if treatment of disease is suspended, and the erroneous assumption that treatment will not change the course of the disease. Both of these are important points, so let's explore them in a bit more detail.

~

Once you become ill, whether you are fighting cancer or some other disease, having a good quality of life generally depends upon controlling the underlying disease. If you don't address your disease, the chance you will achieve a good quality of life is substantially diminished.

Let's consider, for example, a man we'll call Quentin. Quentin has an incurable form of cancer. Together with his family, Quentin contemplates his options for treatment. One of the key points in the family's discussion is that the type of cancer Quentin has is not currently curable. There is a treatment available that offers a chance at remission, but the treatment cannot cure Quentin's cancer and there is no guarantee that remission will be achieved.

Quentin's family is concerned about pursuing treatment because the treatment is likely to be very tough on Quentin, and they do not want Quentin to suffer. Together with Quentin, they have accepted the incurable nature of Quentin's cancer and want him to have a good quality of life for the time he has left. They

---

Ruth's story

Ruth had breast cancer with extensive liver metastases. Once breast cancer spreads extensively in the liver, some doctors consider it to be incurable.

Ruth came to see me. We treated her cancer aggressively. The treatment was difficult and during that time Ruth experienced a poor quality of life. But she eventually achieved complete remission.

Now, nine years later, Ruth is still in remission, and probably cured. And, for the last nine years, she has enjoyed a normal quality of life. She has married a caring man and they look forward to a long life together.

believe aggressive treatment of Quentin's cancer will deprive him of that.

However, Quentin's disease is probably already affecting his quality of life. If his disease is not treated, he will not achieve a good quality of life, even in the short term. Therefore, the goal of giving Quentin quality of life by not pursuing treatment will not be realized.

Further, the treatment, while difficult in the short term, does have a chance of sending Quentin's cancer into remission; and, if it does, Quentin could remain in remission for a prolonged period of time with a near-normal quality of life.

In cases such as this, and really in the case of any disease, there has to be a balance sought between the harms or benefits and limitations or capabilities of treatment. We must face our misconceptions about the possibilities head on. If we believe that it is better to decline treatment and have some quality of life than it is to continue treatment and have a poor quality of life for a short time, we need to consider whether we can reasonably expect to achieve a good quality of life if we don't treat the underlying disease.

We also need to consider all the potential outcomes of treatment. Often, the decision requires weighing the concerns over some level of short-term discomfort against the possibility of a long-term gain in health and well-being.

~

If a patient cannot be cured, and no treatment can impact the natural course of a disease, then the focus can be rightly placed on quality of life. In such cases, hospice care, or palliative care as it is often called, can be an excellent idea. But I believe this is only appropriate when there really is no chance that treating a disease can offer relief, remission or cure, and a patient is truly nearing death.

The problem in cancer medicine is that the chance for remission or cure is not always clear. One doctor may consider a patient incurable, but a different doctor might have another opinion. This can become a quality-of-life issue if you are told by your doctor you are incurable and there is nothing more that can be done for you. In such cases, you may want to consider getting a second opinion or perhaps even more opinions. This is because a different doctor might offer you a new treatment, and while a new treatment may mean a short-term compromise in terms of quality of life, it might offer a chance at survival and a better quality of life in the long-term.

Over the years I have learned, in the context of cancer, one sometimes has to go through hell in order to achieve a positive

Sarah's story

Sarah had nasopharyngeal carcinoma with widespread metastases to distant lymph nodes. Many doctors considered Sarah to be incurable.

I started Sarah on aggressive treatment with a drug she had not received before. The treatment was tough on Sarah and she had a poor quality of life for several months. But we were able to force her cancer into remission.

Today, twelve years later, Sarah's cancer is still in remission, making it probable that she is cured. During these years, she has had a completely normal quality of life.

response. If you and your loved one focus only on the short-term misery and refuse to receive treatment because of that, then you deny yourself the chance to prolong your life, experience remission or perhaps even achieve a cure. And I do not believe anyone should be deprived of the possibility of remission or a cure simply to avoid short-term difficulties. If a treatment offers a real possibility of long-term advantage, then I believe it is an acceptable choice, regardless of its effect on your short-term quality of life.

～

One reason quality of life is such a frequent topic of discussion in cancer medicine and among cancer patients and their families is that cancer treatments can sometimes make patients miserable. But I would hasten to remind you here, they do not always have to be so harsh. Remember, as we discussed in Chapter 9, one of the goals of medical supportive therapy is to improve the cancer patient's quality of life as much as possible. But since medical supportive therapy is often not covered by insurance, cancer patients do not always benefit from as much medical supportive therapy as they need.

If you find yourself in a situation where you are miserable during treatment, and you and your loved ones are contemplating stopping treatment because it seems your treatment is only making you worse, I urge you to talk to your doctor about whether medical supportive therapy could help and what options you have for getting the supportive therapy you need. Of course, medical supportive therapy may not be able to solve every problem, but, if you can get the therapy you need, it might substantially improve your quality of life and prompt you to reconsider your decision about whether to continue treatment. And, as we have discussed, continuing treatment may be all you need to do in order to have a chance at remission or a cure.

~

It is also important to remember quality of life during cancer treatment is not just about physical comfort, mobility and self-reliance. It is also about emotional and psychological well-being. In the context of cancer care, or any serious disease, I believe it is the job of the doctor to instill hope and simultaneously make a conscious effort to not strip a patient of hope. I also believe family and friends can provide the patient with a loving, supportive, hopeful and comfortable environment. For, as we discussed in Chapter 10, hope, love and compassion are vital to your emotional and psychological well-being during treatment and to maintaining a positive outlook. This will improve your quality of life and help you sustain the strength to continue the fight.

~

We have now come to the conclusion of part one of this book, my letter to the cancer patient. Now let's move on to part two and discuss my thoughts on various aspects of medical practice in modern society and the right to health.

PART II

*Essays on Medical Practice
and the Right to Health*

12

THE POWER OF EDUCATION

Education is the most powerful weapon
we can use to change the world....

NELSON MANDELA[1]

I am a great believer in the power of education. Time and time again, education has demonstrated its capacity to revolutionize our understanding of the world around us. Education trains the mind to evaluate data, derive meaning from facts, process new information and make informed choices. Education changes a person from someone limited by what they do not understand, restricted to accepting the direction prescribed by others, to someone who can examine the world around them and participate in determining their own destiny.

In the context of medicine, education transforms our ability to understand health, and to prevent and treat disease. In my years of practice, I have found that, in times of illness, especially in the context of chronic diseases such as cancer, education is a vital part of patient care. Education impacts a patient's understanding of, and outlook on, disease; it permits rational consideration of treatment options and it encourages compliance with long-term treatment plans.

However, patient education cannot take a one-size-fits-all approach. It is important to take into account the intellectual and spiritual framework within which the learner will view the information provided. One aspect of customizing patient education involves considering the patient's foundation of knowledge. Some patients have a good base of knowledge about medicine and health while others have less prior knowledge. For patients with a good fund of knowledge, some topics may be skipped, but if prior knowledge is lacking and educational activities are targeted inappropriately, patients may become confused and the impact of education will be diminished.

Another important aspect of patient education is understanding the cultural, religious and social context within which each patient lives. Every person is different, and patient education must respect the individual not just as a patient, but as a human being.

Throughout this chapter, I offer my insights, gained over many years of medical practice, on various aspects of patient education as it relates to cancer care. I believe this chapter has value, not only for patients, to help you consider what types of information you may wish to get from your doctor, but also for doctors interested in providing their patients with as much information about their disease and its treatment as possible.

~

In my experience, a good place to begin patient education in cancer care is to talk about the patient's diagnosis, including the natural history and pathology of cancer. For example, if a patient has lung cancer, it is important for them to understand there are many different types of lung cancer, and each type of lung cancer behaves differently, is treated differently and responds differently to treatment.

Patients also need to understand the significance of metastasis. For example, if a patient has back pain because of a vertebra affected by metastasis, it is important for the patient to know what this means, recognize that radiation therapy may be required and understand why this is likely to be the best treatment for this type of metastasis. Patients also need to be taught about what to expect, not only from the cancer itself, but also from its treatment. You may recall we talked a bit about thinking ahead in Chapter 4 in the context of preparing for treatment, but it is important to revisit the subject here, in the context of general patient education. Patients need to know about any lifestyle changes that may be required, how medications should be taken, what follow-up is required and what types of problems may occur. Patients need to understand which signs and symptoms are nothing to worry about and which may mean something is wrong. Patients also need to know what to do and who to call in case of a problem.

Additionally, patients need to be educated about the benefits, risks, capabilities and limitations of various treatments for cancer. For example, chemotherapy generally has a bad reputation because it is often given without medical supportive therapy. Patients need to know about the various types of supportive therapy available, what is involved in supportive therapy and how and where to get it.

Other important patient education topics include diet and nutrition, exercise and work. You may recall we discussed diet and nutrition as a component of medical supportive therapy in Chapter 9. But, as a part of patient education, it is often helpful to discuss diet and nutrition in detail, to make sure patients understand that a proper diet is crucial in cancer care, that eating healthy, natural foods throughout treatment is essential and that avoiding canned, artificial or processed foods can be beneficial. Patients also may find it helpful to eat several small meals a day instead of a few large meals, and some patients may need to avoid salt, particularly if treatment includes steroids such as cortisone. Exercise is also important during cancer treatment because it helps patients maintain muscle tone, strength and stamina. Going back to work can help restore a sense of normalcy.

It is also important to keep in mind that patient education is rarely a one-time activity. Often, patient education is more effective when information is provided in small amounts, as it becomes important. Patient education also takes time. It is not usually practical to try to educate patients about all aspects of their disease and treatment in a single session. Patient education must also include plenty of time for questions. The meetings and appointments at the beginning of treatment are excellent opportunities to begin patient education. But patient education typically occurs repeatedly throughout diagnosis and treatment, especially as different aspects of cancer and different treatment options become relevant.

~

Often, cancer patients want to know about alternative treatments. However, the term "alternative treatment" is troublesome because it can be misleading. The word alternative is generally taken to mean a choice between two options. In the case of medical treatment, it may be taken to mean a choice between different treatments: one chooses either treatment "A" or treatment "B", but not both. And while choosing between treatment options is often a part of medical care, the term alternative treatment, as it is used in the United States today, usually means something more problematic. Usually, it means forgoing medical treatments that are proven to be effective, and contained within the accepted practice of medicine, in place of treatments that are not known to be effective and not part of the accepted practice of medicine. Except in the case of well-regulated, review-board approved clinical trial protocols, patients are generally advised against choosing treatments of unknown benefit in place of traditional treatments of proven effectiveness.

In contrast, complementary treatments are not generally considered to be a part of medical practice, but have been shown to have value.[2] Complementary treatments do not interfere with proven medical treatments and are in addition to, not instead of, the medical treatment. For example, chiropractic, homeopathic or faith-based interventions, if important to the patient, and known to be helpful physically, psychologically or spiritually, can have value to patients when used in conjunction with other proven treatments for cancer. Other interventions such as meditation, yoga or other mind-body therapies are also often considered complementary treatments. Although data proving the effectiveness of complementary treatments in the fight against cancer may be lacking, as long as the treatments do not interfere with those treatments known to be effective against cancer, and do not increase the risk of harm to the patient, I generally do not advise against such treatments.

If you are considering complementary treatments, I urge you to talk to your doctor about the various treatments you wish to pursue and discuss which complementary treatments might be helpful and which should be avoided. For example, depending upon other treatments being used, some products such as herbs, supplements or probiotics may be inappropriate, even hazardous, and certain physical activities may be difficult or even dangerous.

~

The objectives of treatment are also an important topic for patient education. Depending upon the type of cancer a patient has, and the stage of that cancer, objectives for treatment may differ. Patients need to understand the objectives of their treatment plan in order to have realistic expectations about outcomes. For example, treatment may be intended to achieve a cure, or it may be intended to relieve pain. When the objective is a cure, it is permissible to push a patient's treatment to severe toxicity. However, it is not typically considered permissible to push a patient's treatment to severe toxicity if the goal is palliation.

An additional objective of treatment is prolonging life. The treatment of cancer is always evolving as new treatments become available. A patient who cannot be cured today, may still be cured eventually if he or she can survive long enough to receive a new drug that may not yet be available.

Quality of life is another important objective of cancer treatment, regardless of the curability of a cancer. For quality-of-life care, patients need medical supportive therapy, hope and compassion. Some may also need psychological therapy. Patients may need to be seen on a regular basis by an internist—and not just any internist: one with expertise in taking care of cancer patients. A seasoned internist, with experience of taking care of cancer patients, brings particular expertise to cancer treatment. This is because patients undergoing treatment for cancer can face a variety of medical issues from time to time, including infections, bleeding, pain, diarrhea or constipation. However, if patients do not understand the value that regular visits to an internist will bring to their quality of life and treatment, patients may not see the need to go to yet another doctor on a regular basis and may not follow through.

~

Finally, educating patients about the power of hope and perseverance is important. Hope fuels perseverance. Perseverance is the determination to continue to go forward. Fighting cancer can be a long, tedious journey. Patients may have emotional highs and lows during treatment, and there may be both progress and setbacks. Some people battling cancer may become frustrated or lose faith, or have thoughts about stopping treatment. But cancer treatment is a means to an end. Perseverance is the drive that will keep you moving, keep you hanging in there, until you reach your objective.

~

Typically, it is not enough to educate only the patient. It is also important to educate the patient's family. I encourage my patients to bring family members to any visits that will involve education, so they can better understand their role in encouraging and supporting their loved one. Family members need to be positive and supportive, and provide warmth and compassion. They need to treat their loved one as normally as possible and avoid pity.

Finally, family members should not keep their loved one in the dark or deny their loved one's autonomy. Family members should also avoid treating the patient as an invalid or outcast, or making their loved one a spectator in their own care. Patients need to be engaged in their care at all times if possible.

~

Unfortunately, there are a variety of obstacles related to patient education. A major obstacle is time. Doctors simply do not have unlimited amounts of time, and time spent on education is not usually reimbursed. In the modern American medical system, where the focus is placed so largely on the financial aspects of medical practice, doctors are often discouraged from spending time on activities that will not be reimbursed.

Some doctors may not be very adept at educating patients. Doctors get plenty of training in medical science and the treatment of disease, but they do not often get much training in the art of educating patients. It takes special skills to translate complex medical information into simple terms that patients can understand. Doctors who lack these skills may be less inclined to spend time educating their patients.

The Internet also poses a challenge to patient education. You may recall that we talked about the Internet as a source of information in Chapter 3, in the context of the group consultation. It is important, however, to reiterate here, in the context of patient education, that there is a lot of high-quality health-related information on the Internet, but there is also a lot of information that is not accurate. It is important that patients seek information online that is written by authoritative sources. Patients also need to be mindful that even information of the highest quality, from the most reliable sources may, at best, be over-simplified or generalized and may only describe a disease or its treatment in broad strokes.

Similarly, information from more traditional media sources, such as magazines, newspapers, radio and TV, may be over-simplified, generalized or inaccurate. As you search for information about your cancer and its treatment, remember that you are unique and even good quality information may not be applicable to you.

Advice from friends can also sometimes be a problem. We also talked a bit about this in Chapter 3, but it is important to remember here that it is human nature for family members, friends and acquaintances to want to share stories and experiences and tell you about what they have learned or, if diagnosed with the same cancer you have, tell you about what worked for them or their loved ones. The information and recommendations others provide can be helpful, and may come from compassion and a desire to be supportive, but the experiences of others may not always be applicable to you.

If you seek out information online or from the media, or receive guidance from family, friends or acquaintances, I urge you to talk to your doctor about the benefits and potential pitfalls of seeking information from various sources. Ask your doctor to direct you to authoritative sources of information, and talk to your doctor about any information you find before you make any decision or take any action based on such information.

In closing, I believe that one of the most important things in caring for cancer patients is to make sure patients maintain a positive attitude and a hopeful outlook. I have found that education is vital in achieving this enlightenment. The power of education gives patients a perspective to manage their disease, comply with and continue treatment, and live a life that is as normal as possible.

Now that you have learned about the power of education in cancer care, let's talk about telling the truth.

13

TELLING THE TRUTH

Truth is the most valuable thing we have.

MARK TWAIN[1]

Telling the truth is essential to the practice of medicine. The truth has meaning. It serves a purpose. It respects patients. It allows patients to understand what is happening to them, participate in decisions about treatment options and assist in their own care. I believe that patients have the right to learn the truth about their disease and its treatment.

Telling the truth is also the foundation of trust. When trust is broken through lies, the doctor-patient relationship is compromised, sometimes beyond repair. It is my belief that a doctor should never, at any point or for any reason, tell a patient a lie.

But I also believe that how a doctor imparts the truth to a patient is just as important as telling it. This is relevant across all specialties of medicine, but especially in cancer care. No matter what the truth is, or how serious it might be, the doctor's job is to always do the utmost to save the life of the patient—and that includes telling the truth.

In this chapter, we will explore in more detail why it is so important that doctors always tell patients the truth about their disease and its treatment, and why sensitivity and compassion are such important parts of telling the truth to patients. I believe these perspectives will help both doctors, as they communicate with their patients, and patients, as they listen to their doctors.

∼

Doctors must tell the truth effectively and constructively, without traumatizing or harming the patient. But achieving this goal requires tact and skill. It is not simply a matter of regurgitating facts and statistics. You may recall that we talked a bit about this in Chapter 10. It is important to reiterate, here, that the problem is not a lack of care on the part of doctors, for most doctors do care. The problem is that, unfortunately, not all doctors are very good at delivering the truth to patients. More likely, they simply have not had much training in the art of telling the truth.

Telling the truth also takes time—time to talk to the patient, explain the facts, and discuss the patient's feelings about the truths that have just been told. In American medicine today, however, the restrictions of payors (i.e. insurance companies) often require doctors and institutions to focus so much on the financial aspects of medical practice that the time spent with patients is reduced. Add in the interference of oversight groups, regulators and institutional reviewers—who require documentation of tasks and completion of checklists, regardless of whether each task is relevant to a particular patient—and the time doctors have to spend with patients is further compromised.

With all of these external pressures, it is easy to see why doctors have limited time to talk to patients. As a result, doctors often do what is fastest and simplest, repeating knowledge and statistics and keeping conversations brief. But this is not usually the best way to talk to a cancer patient, or any patient with a serious disease.

~

Another important element doctors must consider when telling the truth to patients is to personalize the message. You may recall that I described in Chapter 12 how my approach to patient education takes into consideration the foundation of knowledge and the cultural, religious and social context within which each patient lives. These are important attributes for doctors to consider when telling the truth. Every patient is different, and personalizing the message minimizes the chance that the truth is misinterpreted.

Personalizing the message, however, does not mean that I withhold the truth or minimize the seriousness of the truth; it simply means that, in my experience, patients are more receptive to the truth, and respond to it better, when I use words that are understandable and respectful of my patient's cultural and religious identities and social environment.

~

Compassion and sensitivity are also important when telling the truth. When I talk to my patients, I make every effort to tell the truth in a way that does not strip my patient of hope or drive them to despair. Telling the truth without traumatizing someone can be challenging sometimes, but it is something that is central to the ethos of care I deliver to my patients.

Let's consider two scenarios to illustrate this point. First, imagine Tom, a thirty-four-year-old man with melanoma. He has metastatic lesions in his liver and bones. The truth is that Tom has metastatic melanoma and, at present, metastatic melanoma is incurable. Tom's doctor can take two approaches to telling this truth. In one approach, the doctor can tell Tom he has metastatic melanoma which is incurable. But if the conversation stops with the incurable nature of the disease, the conversation could lead Tom to hopelessness and despair. Another approach the doctor could take is to continue the conversation and emphasize to Tom that, although currently incurable, there has been a great deal of progress made in recent years in the treatment of melanoma, and new treatments are available now that may be able to control his disease. If Tom were to choose to take advantage of one of these new treatments, he might be able to prolong his life until a new drug becomes available in the future which could cure his disease. Both approaches tell the truth, but the second approach, in addition to educating Tom about his treatment options, may go a long way to preserving his hope.

Now let's consider Uriel. Uriel has Hodgkin's lymphoma. One approach Uriel's doctor can take is to tell Uriel that Hodgkin's lymphoma is a malignant disease, that he will need chemotherapy and radiation therapy over a long period of time and that there is no guarantee of a cure. Every bit of this information is true, but it may be demoralizing to Uriel. Another approach Uriel's doctor could take is to add that, unlike some other cancers, the treatment of Hodgkin's lymphoma results in a cure in many patients. Both approaches are truthful, but the second approach is much more hopeful.

I am very passionate about this: a doctor must tell the truth and never lie to a patient. But it is equally important to tell the truth in a way that preserves the patient's hope. I believe that the doctor's role is to always try to do what is best for their patient and to never give up on hope, or inflict physical, psychological or emotional harm on a patient.

～

Telling the truth is also a dynamic process. Often, it is not practical or productive to tell patients everything about their disease and its treatment all at once. Telling the truth effectively may require the information be provided gradually, over time.

I am not suggesting that a doctor should ever keep important information from a patient, but patients can be overwhelmed by too much information when it is provided all at once. This is why I recommend that my patients bring a relative or friend with them to appointments. Psychological and emotional issues can come into play that may compromise a patient's ability to hear anything after the diagnosis, or absorb a great deal of information at one time, especially in the context of a serious disease. In such cases, it may not be wise for a doctor to provide so much truth all at once that the patient cannot retain or make sense of what has been discussed, or worse, that the patient misunderstands the information that has been provided. I believe that patients are better served when information is prioritized and given in smaller doses, as it is relevant.

～

Sometimes, test results or other information related to a patient's diagnosis will not make clinical sense. In these cases, it may be best to hold off telling the patient everything there is to know about a suspicious finding until the information can be confirmed.

Victor's story

Victor has pancreatic cancer. Throughout Victor's treatment, I followed the levels of a tumor marker called CA19-9. Initially, Victor's CA19-9 level was 12,000. Over the course of treatment, Victor's CA19-9 tumor marker levels dropped to 8,000, then 6,000, then 4,000. This was a good sign that Victor was doing quite well.

Then, all of a sudden, the next test showed that Victor's CA19-9 tumor marker level was 16,000. This result did not make sense to me. It was out of line with the trend we had been seeing, and there were no clinical indications that Victor was getting sicker—quite the contrary. So, instead of immediately telling Victor everything about this suspicious finding and all that it could mean, I had the test repeated.

As it turned out, there was an error at the testing laboratory. The value that had been reported as 16,000 was incorrect. The result was actually 1,600, a further improvement over previous values. Fortunately, by further investigating this suspicious finding before getting too deep into it with Victor, he was spared the psychological and emotional consequences of what turned out to be an inaccurate "truth".

Again, I am not suggesting the doctor should withhold information from a patient or tell a lie. But, before setting off alarm bells that could cause psychological or emotional harm, or result in very disruptive fear and anxiety, it may be best for a doctor to make sure the information received from a test is accurate before proceeding.

~

For cancer patients, the point of everything we have discussed so far in this chapter is this: if you have questions or concerns about any information your doctor shares with you, talk to your doctor. If you feel that you do not understand something, if you feel overwhelmed or dispirited or if you would just like more time to talk about something, tell your doctor. It is vitally important that you understand the information you are given, that you are confident in that information, and that you feel you have all the information you need at any given time. You may have to advocate for yourself sometimes, but getting clarity on what you have been told and confirmation on anything that is confusing or just doesn't seem right will serve both you and your doctor well moving forward.

If you have concerns about any information that your doctor shares with you, or if there is something your doctor has said that just doesn't seem right, do not be shy about asking your physician how confident he or she is in that information. It may be that the best approach is to confirm the information with a second test or an independent methodology before any action is taken.

~

Finally, it is important to keep in mind the difference between fact and clinical judgment. Facts are based on truth. Let's go back to Tom. The facts are that Tom has metastatic melanoma which is incurable. That is the truth. In contrast, clinical judgment is the doctor's best recommendation about how to proceed in treating Tom. When the doctor advocates for a particular approach to treating Tom's metastatic melanoma, that recommendation is the doctor's opinion.

Sometimes the scientific and clinical data about a disease and its treatment are plentiful, rigorously obtained and consistent. In such cases, the best approach to managing a particular disease may be readily apparent, based on strong evidence and agreed upon as the consensus opinion of experts. However, clear-cut data and consensus opinions are often lacking in medicine.

For many diseases, we simply don't know everything there is to know, and the results of research studies focused on a particular disease or its treatment may be conflicting. Also, research into safer, more effective drugs and procedures is usually ongoing and constantly advancing. So, when data, knowledge and consensus are lacking, doctors generally have to make the best recommendations they can, based on their own knowledge and experience, the most recent clinical and scientific data available and the signs and symptoms a patient is showing.

The problem is that doctors are generally great at expressing their clinical judgment—so great that their opinion can sound a lot like fact. This can make it difficult for a patient to tell the difference between what is fact and what is clinical judgment, but there is a very real difference between the two.

Let's consider a scenario to illustrate this point. Imagine Wilma. Wilma has advanced refractory lymphoma. Most patients with advanced refractory lymphoma will not respond to treatment and will die. But some patients will respond to treatment, and, of those who respond, many will be cured. Wilma's doctor might suggest that there is little point in pursuing treatment because it is unlikely she will respond. But I contend that Wilma's doctor does not have the right to tell her this. Wilma could respond to treatment. She might even be cured. And there may not be any way for Wilma's doctor to know in advance what will happen.

Yvonne's story

Yvonne was told by an expert at a major cancer center that her cancer was incurable and there was no point in continuing treatment.

Yvonne interpreted this information as truth. And while this all may sound like fact, parts of it were really only in her doctor's clinical judgment. Yes, Yvonne had an incurable cancer, but the part about there being no point in continuing treatment was "in this doctor's opinion" only.

Fortunately, Yvonne refused to accept this information. She came to see me and we started her on a different treatment, a treatment to which she responded well. She was not cured of her cancer, but her disease is now under control and she has been living a normal life for eight years, albeit with residual disease.

In Yvonne's case, the doctor did not lie to her. The information he gave her was based on his best clinical judgment, but he did not fully convey her options—it was his clinical opinion that, if she could not be cured, there was no point in treating her further. What he told Yvonne was what he, in good faith, believed to be the appropriate course of action. And while this may have sounded to Yvonne like fact, it was just the doctor's opinion.

This is something else I feel passionate about: I believe it is my job as a doctor to tell my patients the truth and to tell them the statistics, but also to share all of the treatment options available to them, so that we can make decisions together about how to move forward, and do so in a manner that preserves my patients' hope and gives them the best possible chance for survival and cure.

If you are ever in a position where your doctor tells you something very negative, such as that there is nothing more that can be done for you in your cancer treatment, keep in mind that doctors don't know everything. Even if your doctor sounds absolutely certain, and the statements sound like definitive truth, recognize that what your doctor is saying might just be in his or her medical opinion. Ask your doctor why he or she is so certain of the information and what other options might be available to you, including paying for treatments yourself if the problem is that your insurance company will not cover your treatment. You might also want to consider getting other opinions. Remember that a different doctor might have a different opinion. There are often multiple approaches to the treatment of any disease, and different doctors might recommend different approaches for you. Another doctor might recommend continuation of treatment or a different treatment in an effort to control your disease and extend your life long enough to give you a chance to be cured one day.

The point is to make sure you understand the facts you are given. Recognize what represents fact and what is your doctor's clinical judgment, and make sure you are satisfied that the approach to treatment you and your doctor have chosen will give you the best chance for survival and a cure. If you have doubts, consider getting other opinions.

∼

Now, let's move on to talk about the impact of insurance and regulatory oversight on medicine.

14

The Impact of Insurance and Regulatory Oversight on Medicine

You don't train someone for all of those years of medical
school and residency [...] and then have them run a claims-
processing operation for insurance companies.

MALCOLM GLADWELL[1]

But there is no evidence that more regulation makes things better.
The most highly regulated industry in America is commercial banking,
and that didn't save those institutions from making terrible decisions.

WILBUR ROSS[2]

As a physician, I believe it is my perpetual duty to do what is best for my patients, to give them the best possible chance for a cure and do everything I can to save lives. I hold this duty most dear. It forms the basis of my relationship with my patients and is the bedrock of the care I provide.

But the sanctity of the doctor-patient relationship and the quality of health care in America today are under attack from insurers and regulatory oversight entities. The obstructions these groups administer every single day make it increasingly difficult for me to fulfill my duty to my patients.

Insurance companies and government providers of health insurance (payors) interfere with the doctor-patient relationship because they insert themselves into the doctor's decision-making process. For cancer patients, this interference impacts the diagnosis, staging and treatment of cancer. Payors determine which tests, procedures and treatments (i.e. services) they will pay for, regardless of the recommendations of doctors. Payors also set rates for how much they will pay for various services, irrespective of the true costs of the services. As a result, payors exert considerable influence over the services that doctors provide. When the autonomous decision-making ability of doctors is compromised, quality of care is threatened.

Regulatory oversight affects all providers including doctors, nurses, office staff, laboratories, clinics and hospitals. Today, providers must continuously defend their work by documenting compliance with regulations, protocols and benchmarks which have been selected as proxies for quality. To complicate things further, regulatory oversight does not rest with only one group. Multiple groups impose various levels and mechanisms of oversight, and providers must devote ever-increasing amounts of time and manpower to compliance.

As a patient or caregiver, I have no doubt you are aware of the challenges insurance and regulatory oversight pose to your ability to get the care and attention you or your loved one need. Because these are such important problems in health care today, let's discuss them in a bit more detail.

~

Medical care and treatment are expensive. In the United States, we have health insurance to cover some of the costs and minimize the financial impact of illness or injury on individuals and families. In an ideal world, there would be no limit to the financial resources engaged to save the life of a human being. Unfortunately, financial resources are rarely unlimited.

Often, the argument is made that health care is a basic human right and should be provided to everyone without limit or cost. This is economically challenging. It sounds harsh to place a price on a life, but the reality is that health care services cost money and someone has to pay. This truth creates an inherent and clear conflict between the interests of payors and the duty of doctors. Unfortunately, patients often get caught up in the middle of this.

～

To conserve resources, payors create policies that govern the services for which they will pay. Providers must abide by these policies if they wish to be paid. Since patients are responsible for costs that remain after the payor reimburses the provider, failure of a provider to abide by payor policies can leave patients with a big bill they may not be able to afford. In this way, payors influence the decision-making of providers, perhaps not directly, but they do impact treatment decisions nonetheless.

Over time, what happens is that the thought process and behavior of providers changes to align more with what will be reimbursed than with what a doctor thinks should be done. Patients then tend to receive treatment that is based more on what a payor will pay for than on what their doctor thinks is the best possible treatment.

Medicine is not the science of treating a disease, it is the art of treating a human being who has a disease. Doctors know their patients far better than any payor ever could. Doctors are also far more qualified than a payor to make decisions about what their patients need at any given time, and a payor's policies may not always include all services an individual patient will need at any point in their treatment. It would be far better for patients if doctors were able to provide services based solely on what they think is best for the patient, without consideration of whether a payor will pay.

It is important to remember, however, that payors do not have the authority to tell providers or patients what they can or cannot do. You may often hear patients say that they cannot receive a particular service because their payor does not allow it, or hear providers say that they cannot do something for a patient because the payor does not allow it. This is not really accurate. Payors cannot prohibit legal services from qualified providers. All payors can do is say that they will not pay.

If you find yourself in a situation where your doctor feels that you need a particular service, and your payor declines to cover the cost, talk to your doctor about negotiating with your payor. Most providers today have individuals that can advocate on your behalf with your payor. These individuals can assist by writing letters of medical necessity and talking with payors to get coverage for the services you need. You can also advocate for yourself with your payor. You may not always be successful in getting reimbursed for the services you need, but sometimes you will be.

If the appeals to your payor fail, however, you may still have options. Consider talking to your doctor about self-pay options. If you have the financial resources to pay out-of-pocket, your doctor may be able to work with you to arrange the services you need. Your doctor may even be able to work with you on a payment plan if you need financial assistance.

∾

Payors often use standard of care guidelines to assist them in making decisions about what services to cover. Standard of care guidelines generally come from practitioners or medical groups and are typically published in scientific literature. These recommendations name the services that experts believe should be provided to patients with specific diseases.

Many people mistakenly believe that standard of care guidelines represent the best possible treatment for patients with a particular disease, but this is not always so. Instead, standard of care guidelines often represent the minimum set of services that all doctors agree a patient with a particular disease should receive.

As such, standard of care guidelines may not be appropriate for every patient because they rarely take into account the full range of possible services every patient with a particular disease might need, or all of the additional health problems a patient could have that would require services not included within the standard of care guidelines. These exceptions can make deviation from standard of care guidelines the proper course of action, but if a provider performs a non-standard of care service for a patient, a payor may decline payment.

Consider, for example, medical supportive therapy. As you will recall from Chapter 9, medical supportive therapy is important to patients receiving chemotherapy. It controls the complications of cancer and its treatment and makes the quality of life of cancer patients as normal as possible. In my experience, it is particularly difficult to give chemotherapy to a patient without also providing medical supportive therapy.

However, there are no standard of care guidelines for medical supportive therapy because it is so individualized. Without standard of care guidelines, payors do not often recognize or pay for medical supportive therapy. As a result, many patients do not get as much medical supportive therapy as they need. Without sufficient medical supportive therapy, chemotherapy can be very difficult and patients might choose to stop taking, or perhaps never start taking, chemotherapy.

Another concern providers have is that the performance of services not considered in the standard of care guidelines may put the provider at an increased risk of litigation. For example, if a service is available that the doctor feels is appropriate for a patient, but the service is not considered in the standard of care guidelines, the doctor may not offer that service to the patient for fear of being sued if the outcome is not ideal.

Standard of care guidelines often lag behind the science to some degree because they are generally based on published recommendations. New discoveries and updated recommendations take time to filter through into print, and payors often delay paying for the use of new drugs and procedures until they are sufficiently vetted through the process of review and publication. Few would argue against it being reasonable to delay the use of new drugs and procedures until they are proven to be safe and effective, except perhaps in very specific circumstances. However, delaying payment for the use of proven new drugs and procedures for too long can make it difficult for providers to offer patients the most advanced, highest quality, medical care.

~

Some payors will deny claims for services if patients do not get pre-approval from the payor. These pre-approval requirements are an inconvenience and frustration for doctors and patients alike.

They complicate the ability of patients to see the providers of their choice when they choose, and can delay the doctor's ability to provide prompt care.

Payors also attempt to steer patients to selected providers by establishing networks of providers with whom they have payment agreements. If a patient sees an in-network provider, payors generally cover more of the cost than if a patient sees an out-of-network provider, and payors may not pay anything for care delivered by an out-of-network provider. This practice of establishing provider networks often limits the freedom of patients to see the doctors they wish to see, or to choose the clinics and hospitals they wish to use. Provider networks can also change from year to year making it difficult for patients to receive continuous care over time from a particular provider if a payor drops a provider from their network.

~

Another level of control that payors have is determining how much they will pay for services. Services may cost a provider a certain amount, but that may not be what payors want to pay. For example, it may cost a provider three hundred dollars to provide a particular service, but a payor may decide to only pay one hundred dollars for that service. This, in turn, can impact on how much of the cost of the service the patient has to pay. I find this practice of payors troubling, because I do not believe payors have the right to determine how much to pay providers for taking care of their patients.

With regard to physicians, payors often do not pay doctors for time spent on patients when the patient is not physically present. Doctors do a great deal for their patients when patients are not sitting in front of them in the clinic. Doctors review test results, research treatment options, read material sent from consulting physicians, answer questions from patients and perform a variety of other tasks related to patient care without the patient being present. The inability of doctors to bill payors for these services makes it difficult to justify spending time on them. The end result is that doctors spend less time doing these tasks, or refrain from doing them altogether, and this jeopardizes the quality of care patients receive.

∼

Let's move on now to talk about regulatory oversight. Many types of regulatory oversight govern the practice of medicine, including specifying who can prescribe controlled medications, what training is required for an individual to perform various tests and procedures, how laboratories operate and what might bar someone from working in a particular health care setting. We will not talk about these types of regulatory oversight here because they are not so problematic. What I am more concerned with are the recent attempts of oversight groups to regulate every task a doctor performs and how these demands impact the care doctors provide to patients.

What is happening in American medicine today is that a plethora of metrics have been put in place by multiple oversight groups. These metrics often take the form of checklists or surveys and are supposed to measure the quality of care provided. The propagation of these metrics has been rapid and pervasive, and providers have become so immersed in compliance, that they now often pay more attention to computer screens than to patients sitting right in front of them.

Of course, providers have always had to document the care they provide to patients, and it is appropriate that they should. But the problem is that now they are required to do so on so many levels and for so many oversight entities, these tasks represent a substantial burden. This burden reduces the amount of time providers can spend with and on behalf of patients, which in turn compromises the ability of a doctor to address a patient need, and this has the potential to undermine the doctor-patient relationship.

~

Another problem is that some of the metrics used today may be based on assumptions rather than evidence of validity. As the author and newspaper columnist William Bruce Cameron said: "Not everything that can be counted counts and not everything that counts can be counted".[3]

Evidence-based medicine receives a great deal of focus today, but there seems to be less interest in whether evidence supports the validity of the metrics being used to measure health care quality. As a result, some metrics may be little more than time-consuming false surrogates for quality.

For example, hospitals are often required to assess lengths of stay for inpatients and rates of readmission for previously discharged patients. Laboratories are often required to document turnaround time for tests. Intuitively, it seems these measures could have value as quality metrics, but they may not be one-size-fits-all. If relevant variables are not taken into consideration—such as the types of patients a hospital admits, the appropriate length of a hospital stay for each of the various reasons for admission, what caused each readmission or the complexity of tests performed by a laboratory—the metrics may offer misleading information, and providers may be required to implement disruptive changes that will not actually improve care.

~

In conclusion, I believe medicine is an innately human endeavor. The best product America has to offer the world is American medicine. For decades, people have traveled from around the world to get medical treatment here. But I fear the burdens payors and regulators are imposing on American health care providers today are stripping medicine of its humane component, adding further cost, promoting practitioner burnout and deterring the brightest young hearts and minds from pursuing a career in medicine.

Add in the threats posed by the legal system and doctors are becoming increasingly occupied with protecting themselves against the repercussions of not following various sets of rules than they are with doing what is best for their patients.

We need a system where providers are liberated from the constraints of payors, where payors make decisions about coverage based on the expertise and recommendations of providers, where regulators only impose metrics proven to elevate the quality of care and where providers are free to personalize their care to the needs of each individual patient, without fear of punishment or litigation every time they deviate from some generalized protocol.

In such a system, I believe that patients should be free to see the providers they choose to see, when they choose to see them. Doctors should be free to make decisions about what services their patients need without interference, payors should be barred from determining how much providers get paid for specific services, and providers should be accountable for the quality of care they offer but not be held captive by a multitude of metrics and protocols.

There are no easy answers on how we achieve these things and I do not pretend to know the answers. However, I believe we are in this situation in part because of a failure of leadership from physicians to find solutions to the challenges facing medicine. Because of this failure, the will of those outside the profession, outside the doctor-patient relationship, is being forced upon us.

If providers can take back control and gather the best and brightest minds of medicine and economics together for respectful discussions that represent all stakeholders, I believe we can develop a solution that will ensure doctors can practice medicine as they were trained to do, with the everlasting goal of doing what is best for their patients. Providers will be paid fairly for the services they provide, and quality will be measured by the end result achieved for each individual patient.

∼

Now, let's move on and talk about health as a human right.

15

HEALTH AS A HUMAN RIGHT

The right to adequate health care should supersede any other human right.
Even the right to life is meaningless if the right to
adequate health care does not exist.

PHILIP A. SALEM, M.D.

In 1948, the United Nations adopted the Universal Declaration of Human Rights (UDHR). In making its proclamation, the General Assembly of the United Nations declared that human rights are "a common standard of achievement for all peoples and all nations"; and that it is every individual's and the state's responsibility "to promote respect for these rights and freedoms and [...] to secure their universal and effective recognition and observance".[1] In the years since the Declaration was adopted, human rights, and whether governments respect and protect the human rights of their citizens, have become an important political and social driver in international relations.

∾

The primary architect of the UDHR was the philosopher Dr. Charles Malik. At the time he was working on the Declaration, he was also the Lebanese representative to the UN. In later years, he became president of the United Nations General Assembly.

To me, Dr. Malik was much more: a relative and friend, we grew up in the same village in Lebanon. He taught me philosophy. We worked together on political issues and he consulted with me on matters related to his health. I will always have a deep admiration for him because of our personal relationship. I will also forever hold in great esteem his role in the development of the UDHR, because I believe this Declaration was one of the most profound and substantive proclamations ever made by the UN. But, despite my profound regard for my relative and friend, I have, over time, come to the conclusion that it is time for the UN to amend the UDHR.

~

When the Declaration was adopted in 1948, dozens of human rights were enumerated. Among these are:

- The right to life, liberty and security of person
- The right to freedom of thought, conscience, and religion
- The right to freedom of opinion and expression
- The right to a standard of living adequate for the health and well-being of the individual and the individual's family
- The right to education[1]

However, I believe there is an essential human right missing from the Declaration: the right to health. I do not believe the right to health was left out of the UDHR on purpose, rather I believe it was because none of the authors of the Declaration was a physician.

They were philosophers, intellectuals and diplomats.[2] So, perhaps the significance of health, in the context of all other human rights, was simply not fully appreciated.

Article 25 of the Declaration does provide for the right to a "standard of living adequate for the health and well-being of himself and his family, including food, clothing, housing and medical care"[1] but I do not believe this statement includes the right to health, at least not as I define the right to health as a physician. As such, I believe that the UDHR needs to be updated to explicitly include the right to health. In fact, I believe the right to health should be demarcated as the most fundamental human right of all.

~

Why do I believe the right to health should be declared the most fundamental of all human rights? Because health is necessary for life and life is a prerequisite for exercising all other human rights.

Certainly, the rights to freedom of opinion and religion, and all the other rights enumerated by the UN UDHR, are important. But, if you lose your right to freedom of expression, while you lose a lot, you do not lose your life. Without good health, however, you may not continue to live. And, if you are not alive, all of your other human rights lose significance. As such, I believe that all other human rights pale in comparison to the right to health.

~

So what exactly do I mean by the right to health? When I think of the right to health, I think of the right to prevention and treatment of disease. Therefore, I believe the right to health inevitably includes the right to *health care*.

This means every human being has the right to be given access to health care services for prevention of disease where possible, early detection of disease when it occurs and treatment of disease when needed. For individuals, this means that every person should be able to see a doctor for preventive care, have access to health care services when sick and be provided with the knowledge and resources to preserve, protect and restore health. Of course, this is easier said than done, and I do not pretend to know how to achieve access to health care services for every person in the world, but I regard this as a pressing concern.

I believe, if the UN were to amend the UDHR to declare health as the most fundamental of all human rights, the right to health, and consequently the right to health care, would attain immediate and tangible credibility. It would give the issue momentum and incentivize compliance by all the nations of the world. I believe only then will we make the question of how to achieve universal access to health care a global priority. I am hopeful that, with thoughtful attention, mechanisms for providing such services can be devised and implemented.

AFTERWORD

When I was growing up and deciding what I wanted to be, I always knew that I wanted to do something challenging. What made me think of becoming a doctor was my mother. I loved her very much and for many years I watched her suffer with kidney stones. It was because of the relationship I had with my mother, and wanting to relieve her suffering, and the suffering of others like her, that I promised her I would commit myself to studying medicine.

Looking back, I know this was the right decision for me. I cannot imagine any field of study that I could love more. I do not believe anything I could have achieved through the study of any other field would mean more to me than what I have accomplished during my career in medicine, nor could any other profession have given me more fulfillment than I have derived from caring for cancer patients. It has been my honor and privilege to serve my patients, to get to know them and their loved ones, to share in their lives, and to shepherd them through their journeys with cancer.

As you no doubt have discovered by reading this book, I am an ardent advocate for education. Over my years of medical practice and research, I have come to respect the power education has to transform lives. I also understand that knowledge is always in a state of evolution. The more I learn in medicine, the more I realize there are still unanswered questions.

To cancer patients and their caregivers, I say in closing that education is the gateway to informed decision-making. The first part of this book was devoted to you, so that you could learn about cancer and how to gain access to the care and services you need. If I could give you any further advice at the end of this book it would be to never give up the quest for knowledge about your disease and its treatment, and advocate for yourself and your loved ones fervently. My aim in writing this book was to offer you hope and compassion, and to do what I could to give you the best chance for a cure. I hope, after reading this book, that you feel better equipped to achieve these things.

To my physician colleagues, I say in closing that knowledge is the foundation of care, but upon this foundation you must build vision, compassion and love. In the second part of this book, I included you in the discussion of topics relevant to the art and practice of medicine. If I could give you any further advice, it would be to resist becoming discouraged by what you see in terms of the business of health care, keep your focus on what is best for your patients rather than on what is best for your career, and when a patient comes to you and puts his or her life in your hands, dedicate yourself fully to the challenge.

Personally, I have devoted my life to increasing my knowledge, to furthering general medical knowledge, and to taking care of and educating my patients. I have committed myself to being there to discuss my patients' fears, concerns and emotions, and to helping sustain their hope and perseverance. In exchange, I have learned far more from my patients than I have ever learned from any textbook. I wish each of you all the best on your journey with cancer. My love and my prayers are with you.

CITATIONS

1 Diagnosis

1. Hamilton Jordan, *No Such Thing as a Bad Day: A Memoir* (Atlanta: Longstreet Press, 2000).
2. 'Tumor Markers', National Cancer Institute. Available at: http://www.cancer.gov/about-cancer/diagnosis-staging/diagnosis/tumor-markers-fact-sheet.

2 Staging

1. Howard Fabing and Ray Marr, *Fischerisms* (Lancaster: The Science Press Printing Company, 1937).
2. 'Cancer Staging', National Cancer Institute. Available at: http://www.cancer.gov/about-cancer/diagnosis-staging/staging/staging-fact-sheet.
3. 'CT scan', MedlinePlus. Available at: https://www.nlm.nih.gov/medlineplus/ency/article/003330.htm.
4. 'MRI Scans', MedlinePlus. Available at: https://www.nlm.nih.gov/medlineplus/mriscans.html.
5. 'What Is an MRI?', WebMD. Available at: http://www.webmd.com/a-to-z-guides/magnetic-resonance-imaging-mri.
6. 'Bone scan', MedlinePlus. Available at: https://www.nlm.nih.gov/medlineplus/ency/article/003833.htm.
7. 'What Is a Nuclear Bone Scan?', WebMD. Available at: http://www.webmd.com/a-to-z-guides/bone-scan?page=4.
8. 'PET scan', MedlinePlus. Available at: https://www.nlm.nih.gov/medlineplus/ency/article/003827.htm.
9. 'Positron Emission Tomography (PET)', WebMD. Available at: http://www.webmd.com/cancer/lymphoma/positron-emission-tomography.

10. 'Tumor Markers', National Cancer Institute. Available at: http://www.cancer.gov/about-cancer/diagnosis-staging/diagnosis/tumor-markers-fact-sheet.

3 The Group Consultation

1. Keith Sawyer, *Group Genius: The Creative Power of Collaboration* (New York: Basic Books, 2007).

4 Preparing for Treatment

1. William Shakespeare, *Henry V* (London: Penguin, 2015).

5 Surgery: A Medical Oncologist's Perspective

1. William Osler and Thomas McCrae, *Cancer of the Stomach: A Clinical Study* (Philadelphia: P. Blakiston's Son & Co., 1900).
2. 'Sentinel Lymph Node Biopsy', National Cancer Institute. Available at: http://www.cancer.gov/about-cancer/diagnosis-staging/staging/sentinel-node-biopsy-fact-sheet.

6 Radiation Therapy: A Medical Oncologist's Perspective

1. Godfrey N. Hounsfield, 'Computed Medical Imaging' in *Nobel Lectures, Physiology or Medicine 1971-1980* ed. by Jan Lindsten (Singapore: World Scientific Publishing Co., 1992).
2. 'Radiation Therapy for Cancer', National Cancer Institute. Available at: http://www.cancer.gov/about-cancer/treatment/types/radiation-therapy/radiation-fact-sheet.

7 Radiation Therapy: A Radiation Oncologist's Perspective

1. 'Radiation Therapy for Cancer', National Cancer Institute. Available at: https://www.cancer.gov/about-cancer/treatment/types/radiation-therapy/radiation-fact-sheet.
2. 'External Beam Radiation Therapy', American Cancer Society. Available at: http://www.cancer.org/treatment/treatments-and-side-effects/treatment-types/radiation/science-behind-radiation-therapy/how-is-radiation-given-external-beam-radiation.html.
3. 'Stereotactic Radiosurgery (SRS) and Stereotactic Body Radiotherapy

(SBRT)', RadiologyInfo.org. Available at: http://www.radiologyinfo. org/en/info.cfm?pg=stereotactic.

4. 'Immune checkpoint inhibitors to treat cancer', American Cancer Society. Available at: http://www.cancer.org/treatment/treatmentsandsideeffects/treatmenttypes/immunotherapy/cancer-immunotherapy-immune-checkpoint-inhibitors.

8   Systemic Therapy

1. 'Lymph Nodes and Cancer', American Cancer Society. Available at: http://www.cancer.org/cancer/cancerbasics/lymph-nodes-and-cancer.

2. 'Chemotherapy to Treat Cancer', National Cancer Institute. Available at: http://www.cancer.gov/about-cancer/treatment/types/chemotherapy.

3. 'Immunotherapy to Treat Cancer', National Cancer Institute. Available at: http://www.cancer.gov/about-cancer/treatment/types/immunotherapy.

4. 'What is Cancer Immunotherapy?', American Cancer Society. Available at: http://www.cancer.org/treatment/treatmentsandsideeffects/treatmenttypes/immunotherapy/immunotherapy-what-is-immunotherapy.

5. 'Monoclonal antibodies to treat cancer', American Cancer Society. Available at: http://www.cancer.org/treatment/treatmentsandsideeffects/treatmenttypes/immunotherapy/immunotherapy-monoclonal-antibodies.

6. 'Immune checkpoint inhibitors to treat cancer', American Cancer Society. Available at: http://www.cancer.org/treatment/treatmentsandsideeffects/treatmenttypes/immunotherapy/cancer-immunotherapy-immune-checkpoint-inhibitors.

7. 'Biological Therapies for Cancer', National Cancer Institute. Available at: http://www.cancer.gov/about-cancer/treatment/types/immunotherapy/bio-therapies-fact-sheet.

8. 'Non-specific cancer immunotherapies and adjuvants', American Cancer Society. Available at: http://www.cancer.org/treatment/treatmentsandsideeffects/treatmenttypes/immunotherapy/cancer-immunotherapy-nonspecific-immunotherapies.

9. 'Cancer vaccines', American Cancer Society. Available at: http://www.cancer.org/treatment/treatmentsandsideeffects/treatmenttypes/immunotherapy/immunotherapy-cancer-vaccines.

10. 'Hormone Therapy to Treat Cancer', National Cancer Institute. Available at: http://www.cancer.gov/about-cancer/treatment/types/hormone-therapy.

11. 'Targeted Therapy to Treat Cancer', National Cancer Institute. Available at: http://www.cancer.gov/about-cancer/treatment/types/targeted-therapies.

12. 'Precision Medicine in Cancer Treatment', National Cancer Institute. Available at: http://www.cancer.gov/about-cancer/treatment/types/precision-medicine.

13. 'Hormone Therapy for Prostate Cancer', National Cancer Institute. Available at: http://www.cancer.gov/types/prostate/prostate-hormone-therapy-fact-sheet.

14. 'Hormone Therapy for Breast Cancer', National Cancer Institute. Available at: http://www.cancer.gov/types/breast/breast-hormone-therapy-fact-sheet.

15. 'Imatinib Mesylate', National Cancer Institute. Available at: http://www.cancer.gov/about-cancer/treatment/drugs/imatinibmesylate.

16. 'Targeted Therapies for Chronic Myeloid Leukemia', American Cancer Society. Available at: http://www.cancer.org/cancer/leukemia-chronicmyeloidcml/detailedguide/leukemia-chronic-myeloid-myelogenous-treating-targeted-therapies.

17. 'Side Effects of Cancer Treatment', National Cancer Institute. Available at: http://www.cancer.gov/about-cancer/treatment/side-effects.

9   Medical Supportive Therapy

1. 'Think It Through: A Guide to Managing the Benefits and Risks of Medicines', Food and Drug Administration, U.S. Department of Health and Human Services. Available at: https://www.fda.gov/downloads/Drugs/ResourcesForYou/UCM163235.pdf.

2. 'Side Effects of Cancer Treatment', National Cancer Institute. Available at: http://www.cancer.gov/about-cancer/treatment/side-effects.

3. 'Infection and Neutropenia during Cancer Treatment', National Cancer Institute. Available at: http://www.cancer.gov/about-cancer/treatment/side-effects/infection.

4. 'Low white blood cell (neutrophil) counts and the risk of infection', American Cancer Society. Available at: http://www.cancer.org/treatment/treatmentsandsideeffects/physicalsideeffects/infectionsinpeoplewithcancer/infectionsinpeoplewithcancer/infections-in-people-with-cancer-low-w-b-c-and-weak-immune-sys.

5. 'Causes (Germs) and Treatment of Infections in People with Cancer', American Cancer Society. Available at: http://www.cancer.org/treatment/treatmentsandsideeffects/physicalsideeffects/infectionsinpeoplewithcancer/causes--germs--and-treatment-of-infections-in-people-with-cancer.
6. 'Preventing Infections in People with Cancer', American Cancer Society. Available at: http://www.cancer.org/treatment/treatmentsandsideeffects/physicalsideeffects/infectionsinpeoplewithcancer/preventing-infections-in-people-with-cancer.
7. 'Fatigue and Cancer Treatment', National Cancer Institute. Available at: http://www.cancer.gov/about-cancer/treatment/side-effects/fatigue.
8. 'What is Cancer-related Fatigue?', American Cancer Society. Available at: http://www.cancer.org/treatment/treatmentsandsideeffects/physicalsideeffects/fatigue/feeling-tired-vs-cancer-related-fatigue.
9. 'What Causes Cancer-related Fatigue?', American Cancer Society. Available at: http://www.cancer.org/treatment/treatmentsandsideeffects/physicalsideeffects/fatigue/what-causes-cancer-related-fatigue.
10. 'Managing Cancer-related Fatigue', American Cancer Society. Available at: http://www.cancer.org/treatment/treatmentsandsideeffects/physicalsideeffects/fatigue/seven-ways-to-manage-cancer-related-fatigue.
11. 'Anemia and Cancer Treatment', National Cancer Institute. Available at: http://www.cancer.gov/about-cancer/treatment/side-effects/anemia.
12. 'Anemia in People with Cancer', American Cancer Society. Available at: http://www.cancer.org/treatment/treatmentsandsideeffects/physicalsideeffects/anemia/anemia-in-people-with-cancer.
13. 'Pain in People with Cancer', National Cancer Institute. Available at: http://www.cancer.gov/about-cancer/treatment/side-effects/pain.
14. 'Facts About Cancer Pain', American Cancer Society. Available at: http://www.cancer.org/treatment/treatmentsandsideeffects/physicalsideeffects/pain/facts-about-cancer-pain.
15. 'Nausea and Vomiting in People with Cancer', National Cancer Institute. Available at: http://www.cancer.gov/about-cancer/treatment/side-effects/nausea.
16. 'Understanding Nausea and Vomiting', American Cancer Society. Available at: http://www.cancer.org/treatment/treatmentsandsideeffects/

physicalsideeffects/nauseaandvomiting/nauseaandvomiting/nausea-and-vomiting-what-is-it.

17. 'Medicines to prevent and treat nausea and vomiting', American Cancer Society. Available at: http://www.cancer.org/treatment/treatmentsandsideeffects/physicalsideeffects/nauseaandvomiting/nauseaandvomiting/nausea-and-vomiting-nausea-and-vomiting-drugs.

18. 'Non-drug Treatments for Nausea and Vomiting', American Cancer Society. Available at: http://www.cancer.org/treatment/treatmentsandsideeffects/physicalsideeffects/nauseaandvomiting/nauseaandvomiting/nausea-and-vomiting-other-treatments.

19. 'Bleeding and Bruising (Thrombocytopenia) and Cancer Treatment', National Cancer Institute. Available at: http://www.cancer.gov/about-cancer/treatment/side-effects/bleeding-bruising.

20. 'Nutrition in Cancer Care (PDQ®)-Patient Version', National Cancer Institute. Available at: http://www.cancer.gov/about-cancer/treatment/side-effects/appetite-loss/nutrition-pdq.

21. 'Nutrition for the Person with Cancer during Treatment', American Cancer Society. Available at: https://www.cancer.org/treatment/survivorship-during-and-after-treatment/staying-active/nutrition/nutrition-during-treatment.html.

10 The Power of Hope, Perseverance, Love and Compassion

1. Emily Dickinson, '"Hope" is the thing with feathers (314)' in *The Complete Poems* (London: Faber, 2016).

2. Robert Louis Stevenson, *Prayers Written at Vailima* (New York: Charles Scribner's Sons, 1910).

3. Virgil, *Eclogues* translated by H. R. Fairclough (Cambridge, MA: Loeb Classical Library Volumes 63 & 64, Harvard University Press, 1916).

11 Quality of Life

1. Atul Gawande, *Being Mortal: Medicine and What Matters in the End* (New York: Metropolitan Books, 2014).

12 The Power of Education

1. Nelson Mandela, 'Lighting your way to a better future', speech delivered by Nelson Mandela at launch of Mindset Network. Available from

the Nelson Mandela Foundation at: http://db.nelsonmandela.org/speeches/pub_view.asp?pg=item&ItemID=NMS909.

2. 'Complementary, Alternative, or Integrative Health: What's In a Name?', National Center for Complementary and Integrative Health. Available at: https://nccih.nih.gov/health/integrative-health.

13   Telling the Truth

1.   Mark Twain, *Following the Equator: A Journey Around the World* (Hartford, Connecticut: The American Publishing Company, 1897).

14   The Impact of Insurance and Regulatory Oversight on Medicine

1.   Robert Pearl, 'Malcolm Gladwell: Tell People What It's Really Like To Be A Doctor' in *Forbes*, 13 March 2014. Available at: https://www.forbes.com/sites/robertpearl/2014/03/13/malcolm-gladwell-tell-people-what-its-really-like-to-be-a-doctor/#3f0e821e4420.

2.   Katie Benner, 'Mr. Distress is ready to buy' in Top Investor Q&A, Fortune.com 9 March 2010. Available at: http://archive.fortune.com/2010/03/09/pf/funds/wilbur_ross.fortune/index.htm.

3.   William Bruce Cameron, *Informal Sociology: A Casual Introduction to Sociological Thinking* (New York: Random House, 1963).

15   Health as a Human Right

1.   'Universal Declaration of Human Rights', United Nations. Available at: http://www.ohchr.org/EN/UDHR/Documents/UDHR_Translations/eng.pdf.

2.   'History of the Document', United Nations. Available at: http://www.un.org/en/sections/universal-declaration/history-document/.